THE HIDDEN FEELINGS *of* MOTHERHOOD

Coping with Stress, Depression, and Burnout

KATHLEEN A. KENDALL-TACKETT, PH.D.

Foreword by Phyllis Klaus, M.F.T., C.S.W. & Marshall H. Klaus, M.D.

NEW HARBINGER PUBLICATIONS, INC.

Publisher's Note

Distributed in the U.S.A. by Publishers Group West; in Canada by Raincoast Books; in Great Britain by Airlift Book Company, Ltd.; in South Africa by Real Books, Ltd.; in Australia by Boobook; and in New Zealand by Tandem Press.

Copyright © 2001 by   Kathleen Kendall-Tackett
                      New Harbinger Publications, Inc.
                      5674 Shattuck Avenue
                      Oakland, CA 94609

Cover design by Salmon Studios
Edited by Clancy Drake
Text design by Spencer Smith
Cover image: detail from "Breakfast in Bed" by Mary Cassatt

Library of Congress Catalog Card Number: 01-132310
ISBN 1-57224-248-5 Paperback

New Harbinger Publications' Web site address: www.newharbinger.com

02   01   00

10   9   8   7   6   5   4   3   2   1

First printing

This book is dedicated to the memory of my friend
Diane Kay
(1959–2001)
She left this earth much too soon,
but was an example of courage and grace
to all of us who had the privilege to know her

Contents

Foreword

Phyllis Klaus, MFT, CSW, and Marshall Klaus, MD
authors of *Your Amazing Newborn*

The Hidden Feelings of Motherhood by Kathleen Kendall-Tackett is a unique and caring book on the many real issues women face that are sometimes brought on or activated by birth. But this book is about *more* than birth; it is about being a woman in these modern times and about learning to cope with the many unforeseen or unexpected vicissitudes of life and motherhood.

Dr. Kendall-Tackett addresses the enormous load of responsibilities women have to juggle: home, career, infant and child care, and the unrecognized emotional and social changes connected with becoming a mother.

No longer does the home scene resemble the typical family of the *Ozzie and Harriet's* TV show. Today the changing face of the family (single mothers, divorced mothers, older mothers, etc.), as well as the expectations women put on themselves, means that each family is unique. Women need almost superhuman efforts to make it all work.

Not that women haven't always faced rearing children and tending the home, but the demands today and the emotional tenor of expectations often create an overload on the human system that can cause burnout. Dr. Kendall-Tackett not only addresses such important issues facing mothers as isolation, but also discusses unexpected outcomes such as depression, an ill or disabled child, loss, and illness in the mother. She also addresses the difficulties that a history of childhood sexual abuse can cause at birth and the postpartum period.

Dr. Kendall-Tackett not only offers information on what is happening when a woman experiences disturbing events and symptoms, but she also describes some causal factors that contribute to stress. In addition, she gives helpful advice, suggestions, and resources on how to meet these distressing events and circumstances.

She encourages women to recognize that there are solutions; they do not have to do it all themselves; and they are not alone in facing these challenges. Her ideas for self-awareness and self-help, her bibliography of books and sources for support, and her attitude of caring and hope will help many women in this period of their lives.

But let's step back a little. How women are treated and how becoming a mother is understood right from the beginning moments of the birth of her child can have far-reaching implications, especially if she comes home to the more difficult and lonely scene modern women face a few weeks after the baby's birth.

The publication of this book coincides with the discovery of a major principle of the birth process made during recent studies of the perinatal period. This new finding is especially relevant to the major issues discussed by Dr. Kendall-Tackett, since altering the care of mother and infant during this early period can significantly prevent some of these problems.

To fully understand the clinical and theoretical significance of this time (from the beginning of labor, including birth and the next several days), it is necessary that it is identified in biology as a "sensitive period." It is at this time that the mother is unusually open to major changes in her behavior, especially with her infant dependent on how she is cared for during the process. The more the mother is cared for in a humane manner, the more sensitive and caring she will be with her own infant.

Donald Winnicott reported a special mental state of the mother in the perinatal period that involves a greatly increased sensitivity to the needs of her baby. He noted that this state of "primary maternal preoccupation" starts near the end of pregnancy and continues for a few weeks after birth. A mother needs nurturing support and a protected environment to develop and maintain this state. He wrote that only if a mother is sensitized in the way I am describing can she feel herself into her infant's place, and so meet the infant's needs. In the state of "primary maternal preoccupation," the mother is better able to sense and provide what her new infant has signaled. If she senses the needs and responds to them in a sensitive and timely manner, mother and infant establish a pattern of synchronized and mutually rewarding interactions. It is our hypothesis that as the mother-infant pair continues the pattern day after day, the infant more frequently will develop a secure attachment.

Mothers who have continuous emotional and physical support by a doula during labor and birth, compared to control mothers without a doula, are noted in the immediate neonatal period to be significantly less anxious and to have increased self-esteem. At six weeks after birth, the differences in outcome were even greater. Mothers who had a doula during labor had significantly lower scores on a standard test of depression (50% < controls) and lower test scores of state anxiety. They had an easier time managing their infants and began to believe the infant was their own on the third day (while controls first felt their baby was their own on the ninth day of life). They felt the labor was less difficult than expected, while controls felt labor was more difficult than expected. When they were asked to compare their infant with a standard infant, women who had a doula felt their infant was stronger, more beautiful, and healthier than the standard infant, while the control mothers felt their infant was almost as beautiful, almost as strong, and almost as healthy.

Other studies reveal that when the child reaches two months of age, women who have had a doula during labor are significantly more sensitive and appropriate to the signals of their babies compared to women who were randomized during labor to an epidural or a control group. These and other observations suggest that some maternity practices do not fit or meet the biological needs of both mother and infant, are harmful to the young dyad, and may actually be inducing some of the problems Dr. Kendall-Tackett is discussing.

Thus as we closely read the many valuable recommendations for helping mothers suffering from depression, severe stress, burnout, and the birth of an infant with a disability or a premature infant, we also must consider the many humane changes to be made in maternity care. Therefore, we need to look at the continuity and thoughtfulness of care needed at birth and, in addition, to recognize that women in the weeks after birth also need emotional and physical support, practical help and resources, and a culture that values motherhood.

Acknowledgments

There are many people who have given generously of their time to share their experiences and expertise with me. This book would not have been possible without their help.

If writing a book is like having a baby, then these women could be considered the labor assistants. They never knew when a simple "How are you doing?" would result in an earful on whatever topic I had been working on that week. And yet, they continued to ask. My heartfelt thanks to Marcy Alves, Donna Barton, Margaret Jeffers, Marie Goodwin, Mary Beth Magan, Lucie Eldridge, Sue Moulton, Michelle Paquin, Marj Johns, Kathie Martin, and Debbie Rhoades.

In the process of writing a book, sometimes what you really need is a "word in season." These friends spoke encouragement at just the right times, and I am thankful to know them: Martha Vendt, Heather Martin, Annette Dietermann, Nancy Mohrbacher, Ruth Lawrence, Phyllis and Marshall Klaus.

Gerry Koocher, chief psychologist at Children's Hospital in Boston, deserves special thanks for his collegial and generous spirit. His compassion, knowledge, and wisdom are reflected throughout chapters 9 to 11.

Joan Valk and Kathy Whelan both deserve special mention for their invaluable help in the chapter on childbearing loss. They are both examples of grace under the most difficult of circumstances. Mickey Sperlich, and the mothers of the "survivor moms speak out" project, added enormously to the chapter on childhood abuse. I was moved by their willingness to help someone they had never met. Brandi Valentine also allowed me to share some of her story about life with a son with ADHD. I believe that her story will minister to others facing similar circumstances.

Several years ago, Michelle Winkler, former editor of *The Doula* magazine, gave me the idea for the book's title, and acted as a sounding board for many of the ideas reflected in this book. My thinking has also been shaped by conversations with my mom, Pat Kendall, and my friends Maria Tock, Hoke Shirley, Kathy Flannery, Jan Tuxbury, Gerry Ann Dubis, and Ted Cross.

Kate Pennington, Area Coordinator of Leaders in Maine and New Hampshire, offered insightful comments on early versions of my history chapter, and also helped me locate mothers willing to share their stories with me. Many thanks to her and the La Leche League leaders of Maine and New Hampshire (and other places) for their willingness to share their joys and their sorrows. I also thank Cindy Johnson, Lynn Duffy, Paula Oliveira, and the members of the New Hampshire Breastfeeding Promotion Task Force for their suggestions, comments, support, and friendship over the past five years. They have made working in the field of perinatal health a genuine pleasure. My cousin Connie McLennan shared her insights on raising a child with a chronic illness. Her experiences and comments helped shape chapter 10, and by doing so, will help other mothers struggling with similar issues.

I am fortunate to have wonderful colleagues at the Family Research Lab who have offered me an academic home and been enthusiastic and supportive in my work with mothers. I'd especially like to thank David Finkelhor, Glenda Kaufman Kantor, and Murray Straus for their friendship, professional advice, and support for many years. Liza Little has shared her expertise with me on children with disabilities, and has raised my consciousness on an issue that I knew little about. Doreen Cole, who kindly reviewed chapters for me, has also been a faithful ally in the many years we have known each other. I'm always impressed with her wisdom and kindness. Sarah Giacomoni proofed my manuscript and caught all the really embarrassing mistakes that I never seem to see ("we're" vs. "were" vs. "where"). As always, her work was excellent, and she was prompt, cheerful, and a pleasure to work with.

The staff at New Harbinger have been a joy. Patrick Fanning saw the potential of this project when it was little more than a catchy title and half a chapter. Without his encouragement, I probably would not have proceeded. Kristin Beck also provided encouragement at the beginning of this project, and helped me refine my topic. Heather Garnos provided extra hand-holding during the initial editing of the manuscript when I was convinced that I would surely die. I didn't! And speaking of editing, Clancy Drake did an amazing job in trimming, toning, and making it better. She approached her task with tact and humor, and involved me in the process throughout. If you find this manuscript readable, it is largely through her efforts.

My final thanks are to my family. My husband, Doug, remains my greatest and most enthusiastic supporter. He was my in-house technical support, always making sure that my computer was backed up and that the batteries for my laptop were charged. He spent many hours fixing my computer when a certain online provider (starts with an "A") wiped out my operating system. He has also been willing to read drafts (usually with me hovering over him), serve as a sounding board, and generally be a cheerleader throughout. I could never have finished this project without his support.

My sons, Ken and Chris, are the joys of my life. They have taught me what it means to be a mother, and I continue to learn from them. They also gave me the time and space to work, even though it meant that they were essentially "book orphans" for weeks at a time. I am grateful to have them in my life.

INTRODUCTION

In the spring of 1998, I was speaking at a conference on the topic of "Breastfeeding and the Sexual Abuse Survivor." During the break, a young woman approached me. She told me that as a teen, she had been raped by some classmates. She described how this experience had impacted her life, including her relationship with her children. She had never told anyone about the rape or her current struggles.

As someone who has studied family violence for almost twenty years, I have heard many similar stories. But two things struck me: first, I was heartbroken that as a teen she'd had no one to share her terrible secret with; and second, that though mothering was difficult for her, she was doing everything she could to be a good mother.

As I travel across the country, I meet many mothers like her. Some are quite depressed, others are stressed out and miserable. They are tired, and strain under the yoke of too much to do in too little time. One mother told me she hadn't laughed *in years*. What's worse, these mothers think they are the only ones. If you picked up this book, chances are you are facing similar challenges. Mothering is a huge job, with awesome responsibilities, very low pay, and not a lot of respect or support. We all recognize that this is true, yet few of us seem willing to talk about the difficult parts of being a mother. Some of you might simply need encouragement and a few suggestions to get your life back on track, while others may need assistance in making major life changes. In either case, this book can help.

American Mothering: What's Wrong with This Picture?

Do you remember those puzzles where you look at a picture and are asked to circle what's wrong? At first glance, nothing seems wrong, but as you look closer, you start to notice some problems. Well, I find myself looking at American mothers. At first glance, everything seems in order. Other mothers I know seem to function. Mothers in magazines and on TV look good and appear to have their acts together. Yet as I look more closely, I see many mothers who are isolated and quietly suffering. For them, life is joyless drudgery. They think there is no other way. They are stuck.

In response to the time crunch, magazine articles promise to help us use *every minute,* cramming the absolute most into an already too-full day. These articles don't ask whether we actually need to do all the stuff we feel obligated to do. And we are paying a price for our constant overload. I see a troubling rise in stress-related illness—even in children. Then, instead of dealing directly with the causes of stress, we medicate the symptoms away.

Depression is also remarkably common in women in general, and in mothers in particular. Whenever I speak on the subject of depression, I mention how the American Psychological Association's Task Force on Women and Depression identifies being a mother of young children as an independent risk factor for depression—which means it can increase the risk of depression all by itself. That statement always brings a laugh of recognition. But we accept that as "normal," and don't stop to question it. Again I ask, "What's wrong with this picture?"

Who I Am and Why I Wrote This Book

I am the mother of two great sons—and no stranger to mothering stress. I'm writing to you from a wide range of perspectives: mother, wife, scientist, person with a chronic illness, and author of a previous book on depression in new mothers.

In my professional life, I am a researcher in the emerging field of health psychology. I study family violence (especially child sexual abuse), depression in mothers, and breastfeeding. In 1993, I wrote a book for nurses on postpartum depression with Glenda Kaufman Kantor. For the past seven years, I've also been a volunteer breastfeeding counselor. Working directly with hundreds of mothers has allowed me to move outside the ivory tower of academia. This has been a real plus for me, since we research types are not generally known for our "people skills." The idea for this book was first conceived during my many conversations with these mothers.

Though my personal ideals run more toward the alternative or "earth mother," working with so many mothers has given me a perspective beyond my own. I've worked with young moms and older moms, mothers from all different ethnic backgrounds, and moms who are single, who are lesbians, and who range from very wealthy to quite poor.

More recently, my life has taken another turn: I've learned about life with a chronic illness. Four years ago, I was diagnosed with systemic lupus erythematosus (SLE), or lupus, an autoimmune disease that goes through periods of remission and flares. It is unpredictable, and often leaves me with little stamina.

Being ill has forced me to evaluate my role as a mother. Since I have limited energy, I have to make choices, set priorities, and constantly ask which aspects of mothering are truly essential. What is "a good mother," anyway? Why do I sometimes feel bad when I can't be on top of everything the way I "should"? The hard lessons of illness have ultimately improved the quality of my life.

And so it is that I approach the topic of mothering stress, depression, and burnout from all these varied perspectives. Now that you have learned about me, let me walk you through the rest of the book.

An Overview of This Book

The first part of the book (chapters 1 through 3) provides an overview of stress, depression, and burnout. There is substantial overlap between these three conditions, and they share many symptoms. What one person might identify as burnout, another would call depression, and you might find that portions of all three chapters describe events in your life. For you, it is probably less important to have an exact name than it is to recognize the symptoms and learn to deal with them.

The next three chapters (4 through 6) are about one of the biggest sources of stress in your life: work. "Work" includes the work mothers do both inside the home and through paid employment. Because I've discovered that many of the "shoulds" in our lives come directly from our collective past, one of these chapters deals with the history of women's work in America. Understanding these historical and cultural forces helps free us to do what is best for ourselves and our families.

The remaining chapters review some specific issues that might be causing difficulties for you, including fatigue, children with behavior or health issues, and childbearing loss. You can read each of these chapters or just the ones most relevant to your current situation. Each chapter has an overview of the problem and some suggestions on what you can do. A reading list at the end of each chapter gives you information on other publications (including selected Web sites) that may be helpful on the topic. I find that when I'm interested in a topic, I like to read everything I can about it. But since I recognize that your time is limited, I've often provided you with some information about the books on the list, so you can pick and choose. Some of these books are out of print, but you can usually get them from interlibrary loan.

You Can Change Your Life

Your situation may seem hopeless. It is not. Whatever you are struggling with, there is a way out. As you read this book, I want you to recognize the tremendous power that you have: not to change some of your life circumstances, perhaps, but to change how you react to them. Reading that, you may respond that changing how you think only works for people with very easy lives. If you feel that way, you might be interested to know about the life of psychiatrist Victor Frankl. Dr. Frankl, at one point, did have an easy life. And then the Nazis invaded his country. His whole family, including his new wife, perished in the death camps. During his time in a camp, when all vestiges of his previous life were gone, he made a key discovery: that although the Nazis could control all the circumstances of his life, they could not control how he reacted to those circumstances. This power to choose became the central focus of his life's work for the next fifty-two years.

Claudia Panuthos and Cathy Romeo (1984) make a similar point in writing about one of the most extreme forms of mothering stress—the death of a baby. What they say applies to other situations as well:

> No one who has suffered loss is ever again the same; we are either further enlightened and in harmony with our spiritual beliefs, or we are imprisoned in the darkness of our own bitterness, resentment, and self-pity. However

entitled we are to such feelings, they are the spiritual killers of our own souls. Love cannot coexist with bitterness and resentment, nor can we ever grow through self-pity. (xvi)

I'd like to invite you to examine your life. Mothering can be richly rewarding, one of life's great joys. Or it can be an exercise in frustration and despair. You can decide which way it will be for you. Rather than tell you how to cram more into each hour, I want you to be able to live according to your priorities and beliefs. My goal is to encourage and empower you. To help you recognize—and overcome—the hidden feelings of motherhood.

CHAPTER 1

STRESS
MOVING AT THE SPEED OF LIFE

Does your life feel like a treadmill? Do you run out of day before you run out of items on your "to do" list? Do you sometimes snap at people you love? Do you feel you're on call twenty-four hours a day? If you answered "yes" to any of these questions, you are not alone. Even a quick perusal of self-help titles will reveal we are a culture under stress. How many times do you hear the word "stress" in a twenty-four-hour period. How often do *you* use it? When someone asks how you are, do you say "busy," "swamped," "overwhelmed"? Tina, a single mom with three children, says: "I can't cram another hour of 'must do' into my day." If you are feeling like that, rest assured that you *can* live life at a more manageable pace.

A Tale of Two Mothers

Let's take a look at the lives of two mothers. Mary is employed outside the home, while Cindy is home full-time. Mary begins her day at 6:00 A.M. She must shower, dress, and prepare for the day by 6:30, when she starts preparing breakfast. She assembles all the stuff her kids need to take to school, including their snow gear. Do the kids have their lunch money and homework? Are there any permission slips she needs to sign? After the kids are loaded on the bus at 7:00, she hops in the car and heads for the office—just in time to hit traffic. She tears into her office a little after 8:00, only to dash off to a meeting. At the end of the workday, she rushes through traffic to take the kids to lessons or soccer practice. Once home, she begins the nightly ritual of dinner, homework, and chores—that is, if she has no other obligations that night. Maybe there is time to start a load of laundry before dinner. After her nighttime routine, she might try to do some of the work she brought home from the office, or bake the cookies for Jimmy's class party tomorrow. She falls into bed exhausted, only to start again the next day.

Sound familiar? If it does, you know what can happen when part of the plan goes awry: You oversleep your alarm. Or there is no milk. Or the kids miss the bus. Or you spill coffee all over your blouse. Or Tim's mom, who was supposed to drive carpool today, is in bed with the flu—can you take over? Or your child is sick and you also have a tight deadline at work.

Moms at home have stress of their own, as Cindy's story illustrates. Cindy also rises early to begin her day. Her children are young, so there isn't the morning rush to get them out the door for school. But there are plenty of things to do. Tammy was up all night with an ear infection, so Cindy is pretty tired. She calls the pediatrician at 8:00 A.M., but gets his answering service. She'll try again after breakfast. She tries to keep the house clean, but has a hard time keeping up with the messes of three young children and the dog. After a morning outing, she is dismayed to discover that she's just walked through the entire grocery store with a big smudge of food on her shirt.

When she attends a social function with her husband, she is frequently asked, "And what do you do?" When she says that she is at home with her children, the questioner quickly moves on to find someone more "interesting" to talk to. Cindy is very isolated—she's the only mother she knows who is not employed outside the home. By the end of the day, she is starved for conversation with adults. Since she is "not working," others feel free to ask favors: "Would you accept delivery of my package/let the repairman in/pick my sick child up at school/make costumes for the dance recital/bake some cookies/help with the Halloween party?" She enjoys some of these activities; they are some of the perks of being at home with her children. But she'd love a few minutes alone: to take a shower, read more than two pages of a book, or even go to the bathroom. One day it occurs to her that, like her employed counterpart, she has very little control over her schedule and life.

These examples describe basic garden-variety stress—what researchers refer to as "daily hassles." The accumulation of these small stressors can be overwhelming. But let's talk about big stressors for a moment. What if your partner leaves, or becomes very ill, or even dies? Victoria Moran, in her book *Creating a Charmed Life* (1999), describes how her husband died suddenly, leaving her to raise her four-year-old daughter alone. She had committed herself to being an at-home mom. Overnight, her life was turned upside down. Or we might be charging along with life when one of our children gets very sick, or dies. Do we really want to spend this precious time always being on overload? What if you get sick? I can tell you from personal experience that many things change in a family when mom is sick.

Why Mothers Are Stressed

As we enter the twenty-first century, we should recognize that some forms of stress are inherent in our role as mothers, and others are unique to our age. See if any of these common sources of stress sound familiar to you.

Too Much and Too Many

Without even realizing it, we are plagued by the curses of modern society. Stress is often a problem of "too much" or "too many": too many people in a confined space, leading to lines, traffic, and pollution; too much stimulation in the way of advertisements, billboards, and noise; too much stuff and too much time spent acquiring, moving, cleaning, and protecting it. A trip to the post office, grocery store, or department of motor vehicles can take hours and wear us down. Here are some other examples of the stress of "too much."

Driving

We've all heard the joke, "a mother's place is in the car." How true it is! The U.S. Department of Transportation estimates that a person with children travels forty-nine miles per day and that is per person, not per family. Mothers drive children to school, extracurricular activities, and appointments, making an average of 4.3 trips per day. And this number is probably on the low side for many mothers.

Commuting to work is another source of our driving, and our commutes are getting longer. Time spent traveling to work has increased 36 percent since 1983 and commuters spend an average of twenty-one minutes traveling to work (U.S. Department of Transportation 1999). Yet this number drastically underestimates the commute time for workers in more urban areas, where commutes of an hour or more are common.

House

In many parts of the country, housing costs are astronomical, and they dictate many other lifestyle choices, such as the type of job a person takes, the number of hours he or she works, and how far he or she commutes. In areas of the country such as Southern California, New York City, Boston, or Chicago, it is not unusual for a house to cost $350,000, or more. Commutes often expand as families move farther and farther from cities in search of affordable housing.

Housing costs have increased, but so have our expectations. Modern couples often expect to move into a home the size of the house they grew up in, not taking into account that it probably took their parents years to afford such a house. New houses are, on average, twice as large as those built a generation ago, even though the average family is smaller.

Paper

Global paper use has increased more than sixfold since 1950 (Abramovitz and Mattoon 1999). An average person handles about 300 sheets of paper per day. Included in that number are catalogs, magazines, flyers, newspapers, notes, junk mail, faxes, and school papers. In five days, a family of five can deal with 7,000 pages or 45,000 pages a month (Aslett 2000). According to some estimates, we spend an average of eight months of our lives sorting through junk mail alone (Davidson 1991).

Work

Americans work too much. We have recently surpassed the Japanese, and now have the longest work week of any industrialized nation. The number of people with second jobs is at a record high (Armey 1996). We now work the equivalent of eight weeks longer per year than we did in 1969, and we're feeling it. Steven Sauter of the National Institute of Occupational Safety and Health describes the problem this way (cited in McGuire 1999):

> Every day we see reports about the increasing workload shouldered by men and women in this country. Not so long ago we talked calmly about work overload. And then we started to hear the expression "time poverty." Now, at this meeting we're hearing expressions like "time famine."

Time spent at work is time spent away from our families and friends, from our homes, and from self-care rituals such as exercise. Some companies are responding by becoming more "homelike." The net result is that people spend even more time at work (Hochschild 1997).

Debt

Americans are incurring record amounts of debt. The values of thrift and frugality are thought by many to be quaint vestiges from the past. Why wait when you can have it now? This is a philosophy that our country has adopted with a vengeance. The average credit card balance is $7,000, and the average household has ten credit cards. Americans paid $65 billion in interest in 1997 (American Debt Management Services 1998). Consumer credit debt rose from $796 billion in 1990 to $1.4 trillion in 1999—almost double. Similarly, mortgage debt rose from $3.8 trillion in 1990 to $6.4 trillion 1999 (U.S. Census Bureau 2000). Not surprisingly, our savings rate is only 4 percent of our income, in contrast to the Japanese, who save approximately 16 percent of their income (*Affluenza* 2000).

Debt, unfortunately, severely influences families. It dictates how much both mothers and fathers work, and it is a source of chronic stress. Mothers often feel that they have no choice in whether they seek outside employment and they sometimes work two jobs. Families with large debt loads usually have no financial safety net; even those with middle-class lifestyles know they are only one or two paychecks from the street.

The Long Arm of Technology

Modern technology has provided us with items such as cellular telephones, laptop computers, e-mail, and the Internet. No doubt many of these advances have made some aspects of our lives easier. But technology has also increased both our availability for work and the pace of work. Not too long ago, when we left work, we were *gone* (that is, unreachable) until the next day, or the next week. Now, we check our e-mail—even on vacation—and are unwilling to wait even twenty-four hours for information that we can have now. Being "available" twenty-four hours a day has undoubtedly increased our workloads and the pace of our lives.

Vacations

Whenever I travel, I'm amazed at how stressed families are while on vacation. Theoretically, vacations should be times of relaxation and refreshment. But our vacations often take on a more worklike feel. We tend to work right up to the day we leave, then spend a frantic couple of hours packing and preparing the house for our departure. We may drive or fly for hours, and once there, we dash from activity to activity. We return home only to go back to work the next day. Is it any wonder that we often return from vacation more tired than when we left?

The Sum Total of Our Stressors

In *Gracious Living in the New World* (1996), Alexandra Stoddard sums up the malaise of the modern family:

> We are living in a new world, one that challenges our peace of mind and our inner grace. With its frenetic pace and constant state of flux, modern life often feels chaotic and unstable, and leaves us unsure of the ground we walk on. Technology, while providing us many advantages, encourages us to race through our days so that we no longer know what we'd do if we were to slow down. Labor-saving devices seem not only to have failed to enhance the quality of our lives and free up more time, but get between us and the immediate, sensory pleasures of life and increase the pressures on us to do more. Many of us feel cut off from life's blessings, from our neighbors, from the wonders of nature, and from our sense of our own significance in the scheme of things. Modern life leaves us feeling spiritually starved. (xi–xii)

Throughout the remaining chapters in this book, I will discuss many of the issues Stoddard raises. But first, I'd like to describe some of the consequences of the stressed-out life.

The Consequences of Life in the Fast Lane

Of course, a life like this does not come cheaply. If you're living it, you are paying for it with your mental and physical health. A fast-paced lifestyle can negatively affect you, your family, and your community in a number of ways.

Why Stress Is Bad for Us

Much has been written in the past forty years about the consequences of chronic stress. Our bodies have a built-in mechanism to protect us from harm. In response to a perceived threat, our bodies react by pumping out stress hormones such as epinephrine (adrenaline), norepinephrine, and cortisol. This reaction, known as the "fight-or-flight" response, is designed to save our lives in the face of a threat.

The fight-or-flight response is a good thing, but it gets to be a problem when it is constantly activated. Many of the negative consequences of chronic stress are associated with cortisol, one of the hormones your body releases when under stress. Cortisol suppresses the immune system, making you more likely to get sick and stay sick longer. You are more vulnerable to colds and flu, and even more serious illnesses such as cancer. Cortisol inhibits wound healing and can actually increase the amount of time necessary for recovering from surgery. Chronic stress also puts you at risk for diabetes, osteoporosis, heart disease, and hypertension. You may develop eczema or psoriasis. You are more likely to suffer from chronic fatigue. Chronically elevated cortisol can even damage your brain. In sum, it is possible to become very ill when you are always under stress. Your physical health may be affected to the point that you have no choice but to make major life changes.

Chronic stress also has emotional consequences. Ask yourself if being stressed has made you a more cheerful person to be around. Not surprisingly, chronic stress also makes you more vulnerable to depression. There are a number of similarities between the biochemistry of chronic stress and that of depression (see chapter 2).

Unrelieved stress can also eventually have bad effects on your relationships. If you are married, you may find yourself fighting more with your spouse. You may not have time to reconnect with each other and nourish your relationship. In a recent survey by *Working Mother* magazine, 18 percent of respondents wished for more time with their mates, and two-thirds indicated that they didn't have time for sex (Cassidy 1999). But adults are not the only ones who suffer. Stress also affects our kids.

Why Stress Is Bad for Our Kids

Let's face it: when we're stressed, we're simply not as available to meet the needs of others. And though it may not be fashionable to say so, our kids need us. That is not to say we're all they need. But as mothers, we have a unique role—one that is devalued by the culture at large but is important nonetheless. When we are preoccupied with more work than we can possibly do, can we really find out if our kids are being picked on, or that they are struggling with math, or that their teacher yelled at them? Getting to know our kids, or anyone for that matter, takes relaxed time. Spontaneous utterances can occur while we are doing dishes or walking, but they are unlikely to occur during our fifteen minutes of scheduled "quality time."

Family mealtimes also suffer when families are overloaded. Public service announcements plead with parents to try to have one meal together per week. Suburban teens often eat several meals a week at the local mall because family mealtime is rapidly becoming a thing of the past. This is expensive, and has the potential to be hazardous to these children's health.

Why Stress Is Bad for Our Communities and Culture

For a moment, I encourage you to step back and look beyond the needs of your own family. The stressed-out, overbooked lifestyle is also bad for our communities and the environment. To begin with, the stressed-out life is a wasteful one. Have you let food go bad in the refrigerator? Or bought something new because you couldn't figure out where you put the one you already had? Or replaced something you didn't have time to fix? I have. There's nothing wrong with occasionally buying things you already have. What is worrisome is the fallout of a majority of families doing these things on a regular basis. Our buy-and-dump mentality has been having an increasingly negative impact on the environment.

The habits of our culture influence people in other countries. Our demand for cheap, disposable goods fuels some nasty business practices, including the use of sweatshop or even slave labor. Though it is usually impossible to tell whether the goods we are purchasing are made using sweatshop labor, we can decide to stop fueling this market by refusing to adopt the "throwaway" mentality toward our possessions. But it is hard to care properly for our things when we're so very busy and stressed.

When we are overbooked, volunteerism also rapidly declines. Volunteer work is often a logical thing to cut when we have too much to do, but this has an impact on our culture. Schools suffer, for one: parental involvement is directly related to the quality of our schools. For several generations, volunteer labor has held together many charitable organizations; now many of our community organizations have had to stop offering services because there is no one to provide them.

My purpose in outlining some of these problems is not to heap guilt on you, or make you add some things to your endless "to do" list. But I would like you to see that taking steps to reduce the stress in your life is not "selfish." Rather, it is something that can benefit you, your family, and your community.

What You Can Do

In this chapter, I've given you an overview of many causes of stress. Many of the more specific aspects of stress will be described in subsequent chapters, along with techniques for handling them. If you are already overwhelmed, you may not know where to start reducing your stress level. Try to think of it as a journey rather than a sprint. Becoming less stressed may take weeks or even months, but here are a few suggestions that will help right now.

Stop Describing Yourself as "Busy"

When we're swamped, it's easy to tell anyone who will listen that we are very, very busy. As we'll discuss in upcoming chapters, your thoughts are very powerful. Viewing a situation as negative releases the stress hormone cortisol. This is not good for you! Mentally rehearsing your busyness accomplishes nothing positive and is most likely harmful. So stop describing yourself that way. Besides, everyone is busy these days. It's actually fairly boring to hear about the busyness of others.

Guard Your Mind

Be careful about what you allow in your mind. There is way too much information available on almost any subject, and much of it is junk. Pay attention to what you watch, listen to, and read. Even "art" books or films can be excessively negative. Try to be selective and look for material that builds you up and nourishes your spirit.

Do you need to watch as much news as you do, or read the paper, as often? News contains lots of negative information, most of which you can do little about. Many health experts suggest you cut back on how much daily news you take in; Andrew Weil has suggested taking a "news fast." (Having been on a news fast for years, I can tell you that I rarely miss anything important. Really big stories get repeated and talked about.) You can be concerned about the world around you without trying to address every issue. Is there an issue you would like to get involved in? If so, spend your time learning about it rather than trying to cover "all" the news.

Take Care of Your Body

When you're a passenger on an airplane, you are told that in the event of a change in cabin pressure, you should put your mask on first and then assist your children. You can't help them if you are unconscious. A similar principle applies with your day-to-day health. Mothers tend to put others first. While this is admirable in one sense, it is not a good practice in the long run. You cannot strike a balance between your needs and the needs of your family if you are constantly run down. Therefore, you need to consider it a priority to eat well, exercise, sleep, and get regular physicals. Stop getting up early or going to bed late so you can catch up on a few extra chores. If you're going to dig yourself out of stress, then you must stop abusing your body.

Be Unavailable at Least Some Time Every Day

If you want to destress, it is important that you have some time every day, or most days, when you are not available. That means you turn off the pager and the cell phone, ignore the fax and the phone, and don't check your e-mail. It means that you're available when it is time to work, but that you are not available all the time. This is important for at-home moms as well. Have at least some time where you are not available to everyone, even if it means claiming a half hour to yourself in the evening.

Practice Being in the Present

It is amazing how much of our time is devoted to thinking about either the past or the future. Just for fun, make a conscious effort to be in the present. Instead of wolfing down food, think about each bite. Enjoy the texture, the temperature, the flavor. When you're with your kids, practice really listening to them. So often our bodies are there, but our minds are far away. Practice paying attention and enjoying what's going on now.

Plan Restorative Vacations

Give some thought to your leisure time. Are your vacations restorative or do you return from them exhausted? Every family differs in what they enjoy and what they find relaxing, but here are a few guidelines:

- Stay within your budget. There are many inexpensive getaways. Don't add the stress of paying for your trip over the next year (or more).

- Try traveling to someplace closer to home.

- Go somewhere where you can relax too, and don't spend your time cooking and cleaning.

- While at your destination, try to avoid a manic pace of activities.

- Finally, allow a day before your vacation starts to pack and prepare the house. When you return, allow at least a day to unpack and slowly reenter normal life.

Be Grateful for What You Have

Finally, practice being grateful for what you already have. The stressed lifestyle always keeps us looking to what we don't have, what we haven't accomplished, what's wrong with our lives. When we're in the middle of things, it's hard to realize how blessed we really are. How many of us can even fathom what it would be like to have half of our children die before the age of five? Or to spend our days doing nothing but hauling water? Or worry about getting enough to eat? Even if we feel financially strapped, we are most likely materially better off than women in other times or other cultures. Sometimes it's really helpful for us to think about all the things we do have, and to be truly grateful for them.

Another way to cultivate gratitude is to practice looking at your life the way an outsider would. There is a wonderful scene in the movie *While You Were Sleeping*. Lucy, a character whose parents have died, has no living relatives. After saving the life of a stranger, she is taken in by his gregarious family. Over dinner, the family is talking loudly, interrupting each other, not saying anything particularly brilliant. Yet Lucy is drinking in the entire scene. Rather than thinking that this family is annoying, she is glad to be part of it, even if only on a temporary basis. By standing back and looking at your life, you may start to see the things that are really going well for you.

For Further Reading

There are many wonderful books written for people who want to do something about the stress in their lives, or who just want to slow down and simplify their lives Below are a few of my favorites.

Resources for Stress

Bodger, C. 1999. *The Smart Guide to Relieving Stress.* New York: John Wiley & Sons.

Lewis, D. S., with G. Lewis. 1989. *Motherhood Stress: Finding Encouragement in the Ultimate Helping Profession.* Dallas: Word. This book is unfortunately out of print, but you can probably find it through interlibrary loan.

Rogak, L. 1999. *The Smart Guide to Managing Your Time.* New York: John Wiley & Sons.

National Library of Medicine/National Institutes of Health: www.nlm.nih.gov/medlineplus/stress

Stop Stress: www.stopstress.com

Stress Virtual Library: www.clas.ufl.edu

Resources for Simplifying Life

Davidson, J. 1991. *Breathing Space: Living and Working at a Comfortable Pace in a Sped-Up Society.* New York: MasterMedia.

St. James, E. 1999. *Living the Simple Life: A Guide to Scaling Down and Enjoying More.* New York: Hyperion.

Wright, H. N. 1998. *Simplify Your Life: And Get More Out of It!* Wheaton, Ill: Tyndale.

Organized Home: www.organizedhome.com

Real Simple magazine: subscribe at www.realsimple.com

CHAPTER 2

DEPRESSION
LIFE WITHOUT JOY

Is life difficult for you most days? Do you find that you feel sad most of the time? Or do you feel empty and numb? Are things that you used to enjoy no longer fun? If any of this sounds like you, you may be suffering from depression. Depression happens to lots of people, and occurs so often that it is frequently called the "common cold" of mental illnesses. Throughout their lives, women are twice as likely as men to suffer from depression. And mothers of young children are particularly vulnerable (McGrath et al. 1990).

Why Do Mothers Get Depressed?

Why are women especially vulnerable to depression? This is a question that has intrigued researchers. In the popular press, "hormones" often get the blame. But the research literature shows this is a truly inadequate explanation. For example, if hormonal fluctuations were to blame for depression, why does the percentage of depressed mothers continue to increase throughout the first postpartum year rather than only in the early days after a baby's birth, when hormones fluctuate dramatically? Hormones alone also cannot explain why a mother of school-age children might become depressed. There are often very good reasons why women become depressed, reasons having to do with the circumstances of their lives.

In chapter 1, I described some of the factors that can contribute to stress: feeling out of control of your life; always feeling like there are more tasks than there are hours in a day. These feelings, especially when they are persistent, can also contribute to depression. But depression can be associated with a myriad of other factors including fatigue, traumatic events, lack of confidence in your own mothering ability, and lack of help and support from others in your life. Causes of depression vary from woman to woman; what causes one woman to be depressed may not affect another woman at all.

The following pages outline some broad categories of events and circumstances that can lead to or aggravate depression. This is by no means a complete list, but it is a good starting place. Discussions of more specific causes of depression are woven throughout the remaining chapters of this book.

Violence Against Women

Violence is perhaps the most potent pathogen to women's mental health, and it remains a fact of life for many. It can impact every aspect of a woman's life, including her current relationship with her partner and her children.

Approximately one in five women in the general population has experienced child sexual abuse. And while sexual abuse has been studied most often, it is not the most common type of child abuse. According to the Third National Incidence Study of Child Abuse and Neglect, both physical abuse and child neglect are even more common (Sedlak and Broadhurst 1996). The problem of violence against women doesn't end in childhood. Women continue to be vulnerable to rape and domestic abuse throughout their lives. Those who have experienced childhood abuse are even more likely to be revictimized, either through sexual assault or domestic abuse.

Depression is a common effect of past and current abuse. For example, Briere and Elliot (1994) estimate that depression is four times more likely among adult survivors of childhood sexual abuse than it is among the general population. More recent studies on physical abuse suggest similar results. These effects are described in chapter 8.

COST OF DEPRESSION

In a recent survey by the World Health Organization, researchers found that while depression had little direct impact on death rates worldwide, it accounted for 28 percent of all disability (Holden 2000).

Poverty

The American Psychological Association's Task Force on Women and Depression has also identified poverty as a risk factor for depression in women (McGrath et al. 1990). Much has been written in recent years about the "feminization of poverty," or the fact that women are more likely than men to be poor. Interestingly, women who are survivors of childhood abuse are at increased risk for living in poverty (Amundson 2000). Single mothers raising children are especially likely to be poor; such families are both the fastest growing group of our nation's poor (Scoon-Rogers 1999) and also comprise the majority (55 percent) of poor families (U.S. Census Bureau 1998a). And this is not simply a problem of being a single parent: female-headed households have twice the poverty rate of custodial fathers (Scoon-Rogers 1999).

There are many problems related to poverty. Poor women tend to have fewer resources available, and less support. They may live in neighborhoods that are unsafe. They may worry about their children's safety at day care or school. They may constantly worry whether child support payments will arrive. In a recent study examining factors related to "nervous breakdowns," women most at risk were poor, young, single mothers with no religious affiliation (Swindle et al. 2000).

Middle-class women may become poor once they divorce. They may need to move from their homes, and face new worries about making ends meet. In one recent study, women whose income didn't drop after a divorce were less depressed, more positive in their interactions with their children and less authoritarian in their discipline style than were women whose divorce put them in poverty. The children of families with adequate financial resources also fared better socially, behaviorally, and cognitively. The authors speculate that the children did better because their mothers were less likely to be depressed (Murray 2000).

Fatigue and Sleep Deprivation

Sleep deprivation can wreak havoc on a woman's emotional state. Perhaps because it is so common, its influence on a mother's mental health is often overlooked. A little-known fact is that some children do not consistently sleep through the night *for years*. Mothers often do not advertise their children's sleep patterns to others because sleeping through the night is regarded as a sign of good parenting. To admit their children do not sleep well is to invite criticism. Even when kids are sleeping through the night, mothers may be using this time to catch up on chores. Sleep deprivation is widespread and has alarming effects on our health and the health of others. Sleep deprivation and fatigue are described in more detail in chapter 7.

Loss

Hundreds of thousands of women suffer significant losses each year. These losses take many forms: childbearing loss, loss associated with a less-than-perfect birth or a sick child, and mothering in the wake of past abuse—dealing with our own lost childhoods or lost selves. And yet, women are often not given a chance to grieve, or even acknowledge these losses. Within a very short period of time, they are expected to "get on with it."

In upcoming chapters, we will talk about several different types of loss.

Social Isolation or Lack of Social Support

Women who have good support are significantly less likely to become depressed than women who don't. Study after study has confirmed this, and we know it's true. But often our overbooked lifestyles drive away the support we need. In a recent survey in *Working Mother* magazine, "time with husband" and "time with friends" were very often missing from reader's schedules (Cassidy 1999).

Isolation can be a particular problem for mothers at home with small children, or those who are the only ones home during the day. Many mothers live in rural locations and are isolated by geography, some without a car or access to public transit. Sometimes too, mothers become isolated from each other because we fear judgment. Other mothers can be our harshest critics. And we anticipate that criticism and don't ask each other for help.

Husbands and partners can be significant sources of support. Other times, mothers carry the responsibility for the emotional and physical health of their families all alone. Marianne describes how the many responsibilities that she carried alone contributed to her depression. Her battle with depression began after a series of sleepless nights:

> My husband is a self-employed home builder. Under financial pressure, he had to let his secretary and worker go. He had all the calls from his business directed to the

house. My husband was building three large speculative homes, and I was the decorator. We had also started to home-school our five-year-old and I was nursing a baby. I had baby-sitting for two hours a week, and that's when I would make all these big decorating decisions. I felt like the success of these three expensive homes was on me, and I stopped sleeping at night.

All the above factors and more can contribute to depression. If you are depressed, it's important that you understand depression and know what your treatment options are. The next section gives an overview of depression; the section after that suggests what you can do.

Depression: An Illness of Body and Mind

Depression is an illness that affects both body and mind. Both physiology and the circumstances of our lives contribute to it. Depression could be viewed as an emotional alarm bell that lets you know when something is not right in your life. The underlying cause could be something as straightforward as sleep deprivation, or as complex as a history of childhood trauma.

"Better Living Through Chemistry"

One of the giant chemical companies has presented their products as "better living through chemistry." We Americans seem to take a similar approach to depression, which is often described as being due to a "chemical imbalance." The solution that is usually offered to "fix" the chemical imbalance is medication. While it is true that there *is* a chemical imbalance in depression, this answer is incomplete.

Our best biological theory of depression is that it is due to low levels of the neurotransmitter serotonin in the brain. Generally, medications that increase levels of serotonin decrease depression. The newest class of antidepressants—the selective serotonin reuptake inhibitors (SSRIs)—specifically target serotonin. Examples of SSRIs include Prozac, Zoloft, Paxil, and Celexa.

The serotonin explanation seems to be true a majority of the time, but the picture is actually much more complex. For example, we know that some effective antidepressants influence levels of neurotransmitters other than serotonin. If depression was solely related to serotonin levels, why would these medications work? We also know that some antidepressants actually *lower* serotonin levels and still work as antidepressants. And there are at least fifteen different kinds of serotonin receptors that we have identified so far. The effectiveness of these various medications also seems related to which type of receptor they work with.

Another biological aspect of depression is the elevated level of the stress hormone cortisol in people who are depressed, especially those with major depression. The relationship between serotonin and cortisol levels is not fully understood, but it appears that serotonin helps regulate cortisol. As we discussed in the last chapter, chronically elevated cortisol levels cause all kinds of mischief in the body. Depression also seems to leave a biological "mark" on the body that makes people more vulnerable to future stressors, leading to another bout with depression.

An alternative way of looking at depression is to consider it an illness of both body and mind. The chemical-imbalance perspective is that the body influences the mind. But this is a two-way street. Our biochemistry can influence our emotional state, and our thoughts, behaviors, and experiences can influence the biochemistry of our brains. What this means, in practical terms, is that there are other things you can do to create favorable changes in the biochemistry of your brain. For example, both exercise and carbohydrates can increase serotonin levels. And when you think negatively about a situation or event, your body releases cortisol. Thus a tendency to look at things in a negative way increases your susceptibility to depression.

Why Depression Is Harmful

When you are in the midst of depression, it is often difficult to think about how depression can be harmful. But it hurts both you and your family.

Why Depression Is Bad for You

Let's start with you. Besides making you miserable, depression can be very bad for your health. This has to do with the effects of chronically elevated levels of the stress hormone cortisol. By elevating cortisol levels, depression suppresses the immune system (Weisse 1992). You have fewer white blood cells, and the ones you have are less effective in protecting you from pathogens (Avissar et al. 1997). If you have ever taken cortisone-based medications (e.g., prednisone), you know that they are prescribed to temper an overactive immune system, as in the case of allergies, asthma, or autoimmune disease. Naturally occurring cortisol does the same thing.

Depression also has some unexpected long-term effects. Stress and illness researcher Robert Sapolsky (1996) noted that depression can lead to atrophy of a structure in the brain called the hippocampus, which is related to learning and memory. Again, cortisol is the culprit. A question that is concerning researchers who study depression is whether it increases the likelihood of Alzheimer's or other memory-related diseases.

Why Depression Is Bad for Your Family

When you are depressed, you are not the only one who suffers. When one or both partners are depressed, it can sour a relationship and break up a marriage. You may find yourself withdrawing from others who can offer help and support. Or others may withdraw from you. Depressed people can be irritable and critical, and generally not much fun to be around.

But the most insidious effects may be on your children. Depression can influence the way you interact with your children and many problems children have are related to these interactions. Hundreds of studies have demonstrated the negative effects on babies and children of having a chronically depressed mother. It can influence their brain development and lower their IQ. It can impact their relationships with peers and make them more prone to depression (National Institute of Child Health and Human Development 1999).

Researchers have noted that depressed mothers interact in one of two styles: avoidant or angry-intrusive. Mothers with an avoidant style spend most of their time disengaged from their babies or children. They often do not make eye contact and they are oblivious to their children's cues. Mothers with an angry-instrusive style spend more time interacting with their children, but their interactions are tinged with anger and resentment. Both of these styles raise cortisol levels in the children, and these effects have been measured even in babies (Radke-Yarrow 1998).

I'm not trying to make you feel guilty about being depressed. Chances are you've been doing this to yourself. Also understand that it's unlikely you've irreparably harmed your children. Fortunately, children are resilient and do not require perfect parenting. I do, however, passionately want to persuade you to take your depression seriously. Sometimes, mothers believe that they are being selfish if they take some time to nurture themselves and limit their obligations. But this type of self-care is essential for your health and the well-being of your family.

What You Can Do

Fortunately, there are many steps you can take to feel better. Available treatments include cognitive therapy, nutrition, supplements, exercise, herbs, and antidepressants. I've outlined these below, and also included an extensive reading list for further information.

Resolve to Do Whatever It Takes to Get Better

Your first step toward getting better is to decide you are no longer willing to be depressed. This resolve is necessary, because it may take some trial and error before you find a solution that works for you. Even medications don't automatically work for everyone who tries them, and may take several tries before you and your doctor find the right dosage or combination. Realizing that treatment for depression is not instantaneous gives you a greater chance of success.

Rule Out Physical Causes

It is a good idea to have a physical as you begin treatment for depression. Depression can sometimes be caused by anemia or low thyroid levels. Some basic blood tests can rule these causes out. Since sleep deprivation can trigger depression, you might also start paying attention to your sleeping habits. Try to get a good night's sleep: set regular sleeping times (if possible); try to relax in the hour or so before you go to bed; try not to exercise or drink caffeine in the evening; and be careful about the amount of alcohol you consume before bed. For more information on establishing good sleeping habits, see chapter 7.

Know Your Treatment Options

Our knowledge of how to treat depression has grown significantly over the past twenty years. You have lots of options, especially if you have mild to moderate depression. I've listed several options below, which you can either combine or use one at a time. **If your depression is so severe that you cannot function or get out of bed, or you are thinking of killing yourself, or feel that your depression**

is getting worse, please see your doctor right away. You will probably need to be on medication. However, you can also use some of
these other approaches as adjuncts to your treatment.

Good Nutrition

The first foundation of good mental health is good nutrition.
Naturopathic doctors such as Michael Murray (1996) emphasize a
balanced diet as a good foundation for treatment of depression. This
diet should be low in fat, refined sugar, and caffeine and high in vegetables, fruits, and whole grains.

Another nutritional alternative involves carbohydrates intake.
According to MIT researcher Judith Wurtman, your brain needs carbohydrates to make serotonin, and eating forty-five grams of carbohydrates with little or no fat, and with no protein for at least an hour,
has an antidepressant effect. If you are interested in trying this
approach, you might want to get her book *The Serotonin Solution*
(1997). This is a diet book, but she has a very interesting discussion of
the multiple functions of serotonin. She also has a diet plan specifically for "Stressed Moms."

Supplements

Like good nutrition itself, nutritional supplements help form a
good foundation for mental health. Women who are depressed are
frequently low in B6, B12, folic acid, choline, and omega-3 fatty acids,
and supplementing these nutrients is helpful in alleviating depression.

Exercise

Exercise is also an effective treatment for depression. Daily
physical exercise boosts mood by increasing levels of the
neurotransmitters serotonin and dopamine, and by releasing
endorphins. Endorphins relieve pain and create a sense of well-being;
they tend to be low in people who are depressed. Twenty to sixty
minutes of walking or other activity, even strength training, can help
your mood by creating the very chemical changes that medications
create. Exercise can also be an important adjunct to other treatments.
One of the best home programs I've found is *Strong Women Stay
Young* by Miriam Nelson (1998). This book outlines an exercise program used in a study at Tufts University on women in their sixties,
seventies, and even eighties. Nelson, herself a mother of three young
children, offers wonderful support and advice on how to fit strength

training into your life. This very workable exercise program is helpful no matter what your current fitness level.

Cognitive-Behavioral Therapy

Cognitive-behavioral therapy is a highly effective treatment for depression, and is one of the only "talk therapies" that is as effective as medication for treatment of depression, anxiety, and a host of other conditions. Its central premise is that depression is caused by distortions in thinking. It is *not* about replacing negative thoughts with "happy" ones. Rather, it is a technique that helps you identify patterns of negative thoughts and asks you to judge whether these thoughts are *true*. In the book *Feeling Good* (1999), psychiatrist David Burns identifies ten types of cognitive distortions including:

- **All-or-nothing thinking.** Seeing things in black-or-white categories. If a situation falls short of perfect, you see it as a "total failure."

- **Overgeneralization.** Thinking that one mistake changes everything. Whenever you use words like "always" or "never," you may be thinking in this way.

- **"Should" statements.** Unrealistic expectations you may have for yourself and others.

Cognitive therapy helps people identify these distortions and replace them with more accurate (and less self-defeating) cognitions. If you want to try cognitive therapy, I highly recommend *Feeling Good: The New Mood Therapy* (1999). You can also find a therapist who practices cognitive therapy through your state psychological association, or through David Burns' Web site (www.feelinggood.com).

Herbs

Herbal antidepressants have been enjoying a surge of popularity in the United States. Many people are attracted to them because they are natural, frequently cheaper than prescription medications, and generally have fewer side effects. People also like being able to take them without a prescription, thereby exercising more control over their own mental healthcare. (Many physicians are uncomfortable with patients self-medicating, however.) Bear in mind that, natural or not, these substances are medications, and should be used judiciously. Tell your healthcare provider if you are taking herbs and be very cautious about mixing them with prescription medications.

Also, because herbal medications are gentler than prescription medications, they may take longer to work. Be sure to allow at least two months before you decide whether these medications are working for you.

St. John's Wort. The most widely used of the herbal antidepressants is St. John's Wort (SJW). SJW is safe and effective, and takes about four to six weeks to alleviate mild to moderate depression. It has been shown to be as effective as tricyclic antidepressants in numerous clinical trials, without the side effects (Murray 1996). It should not be used for severe depression. SJW is also used for stress and pain, to help with menopausal symptoms, and as an external remedy for wounds, bruises, and burns (Khalsa 2000).

For breastfeeding mothers, the reports are mixed as to whether it is safe. Pharmocologist Thomas Hale (1999) feels we don't know enough about this medication to assume it is safe for breastfeeding mothers. On the other hand, the *German Commission E Monographs* (Blumenthal 1996) the manual used by the national health program of Germany, lists SJW as safe for both pregnancy and lactation.

Some have expressed concern that SJW is a MAO inhibitor (see below) and it has been shown to be function in this way in mice, but not in humans. Patients who take MAO inhibitors cannot eat or drink anything with tyramine, a compound in aged foods. Yet SJW is widely used in France without dietary restrictions, and the French consume large amounts of cheese and red wine, both of which contain tyramine.

SAM-e. (s-adrenosyl-methionine). SAM-e is made in the human body from the amino acid methionine. It eases depression by producing serotonin and dopamine. Interestingly, our bodies' manufacturing of this substance is impaired if we are low in vitamins B6, B12, and folic acid. These same substances are also low in people who are depressed. SAM-e is widely used in Italy and Germany for both depression and arthritis. Unlike other antidepressants, it works within one week. Its one drawback is that it can be expensive, and is often not covered by insurance. Its effects on breastfeeding are also unknown.

Antidepressants

The final option for the treatment of depression is antidepressant medication. There are basically three types. All work to increase the amount of neurotransmitters (serotonin, norepinephrine, or dopamine) available in the brain.

Tricyclics. The tricyclics are the oldest, and cheapest, antidepressants. They include medications such as Pamelor (nortriptyline) and Elavil (amitriptyline). They are often effective, but tend to have side effects such as dry mouth and constipation.

Monoamine Oxidase (MAO) Inhibitors. These antidepressants are also very effective, but when taking them, you cannot eat or drink anything with tyramine. Tyramine is in common foods such as red wine and cheese. When these are consumed with a MAO inhibitor, heart attack or death can occur. These are not widely used in this country, but may be prescribed if other types have failed.

Selective Serotonin Reuptake Inhibitors (SSRIs). SSRIs are the newest class of antidepressants, and include such well-known medications as Prozac, Zoloft, Paxil, and Celexa. As their name implies, they work specifically on serotonin receptors. While these medications still have side effects, they have fewer than the other antidepressants, and their dosing schedule is less complex.

Deciding Whether to Take Medications

The decision about whether to take medications is very personal. If you decide to use medication, it does not mean that you have "failed," or that you are weak. I always feel bad when mothers tell me that none of the other techniques worked for them, so now they'll try medication. You do not need to run through all the other treatment options before you "earn the right" to be on medications. On the other hand, I've also spoken with mothers who had strong feelings against medication and felt forced by their doctor or their family members to take antidepressants.

Please always remember that this is your decision. You are the one who lives in your body, and who lives your life. My role, and the role of any healthcare provider, is to provide information and help you weigh the pros and cons of medication use. Consider the type of symptoms you have: medications help treat sleep disturbance, especially early morning or frequent awakening that is not related to child care; appetite disturbance, (eating too much or too little); fatigue; decreased sex drive; restlessness or agitation; impaired concentration; and "pronounced anhedonia," or the inability to experience any type of pleasure (Preston and Johnson 1997). If your depression is severe and/or you have these types of symptoms, medications may be the best approach. Two very helpful books are *Feeling Good* by David Burns (1999) and *When Words Are Not Enough* (1997) by Valerie Raskin.

Melissa describes how medications took awhile to work for her, but eventually helped get her life back on track:

I'm still on Pamelor. My doctor altered my dosage so it's now triple what he started me on. It took about a month to feel any effects, but for about a month and a half now I have felt great. I'm convinced the medication is helping. I feel I can look a little more objectively at the past year and tell it really was something out of my control to fix, and I wasn't doing it to myself. I'm so grateful to be feeling over the hump. I don't expect a bed of roses but at least life is starting to be fun again. I'm glad I went ahead with medication. I hope and pray I don't ever have to face depression again.

Medications are also probably called for if you have a history of depression that was successfully treated with antidepressants. That medication will probably work for you again. Similarly, if you have a history of bipolar depression ("manic depression"), medications are called for.

Special Considerations for the Breastfeeding Mother

Often, when women are breastfeeding, they are concerned about using medications. Sometimes women will either wean before they want to, or refuse to take medications that may be necessary in their treatment. Fortunately, these are not the only two choices. It is possible to take medications safely while breastfeeding. You do need to know when the level of medication is likely to peak in your milk, and how the medication is metabolized. If the parts that the medication breaks down into are active (called "active metabolites"), there will be more of it in your milk. If the medication has inactive metabolites there will be significantly less of it in your milk. Among the SSRIs, Prozac and Celexa both have active metabolites. Paxil and Zoloft do not, so are preferable for a breastfeeding mother.

"Medication peak" refers to the time between when you took the medication to when it is at the highest level in your milk. The peak times for several popular medications are: Paxil, 4 hours; Zoloft, 7 to 8 hours; Elavil, 2 to 4 hours; Pamelor, 7 to 8.5 hours; and Toranil, 1 to 2 hours. You will need to avoid breastfeeding during this time. However, you do not need to pump your milk to get rid of the medication; it is reabsorbed back into your body. For more information, refer to Thomas Hale's *Medications and Mothers' Milk* (1999). This book is updated every year, so if you have questions you might want to get a copy, or log onto his Web site.

Some Final Thoughts

You do not need to feel helpless in the face of depression. There are many options available to you. My prayer is that you will find the technique or combination of techniques that works well for you. You are worth it!

For Further Reading

Resources for Depression and Antidepressant Medication

Burns, D. 1999. *Feeling Good: The New Mood Therapy.* New York: Avon. Approximately 40 percent of Dr. Burns' patients take medications in addition to cognitive therapy. He weighs the pros and cons of medications, and also provides a very complete listing of medications, side effects, and drug interactions.

Hale, T. W. 1999. *Medications and Mothers' Milk.* Amarillo, Tex.: Pharmasoft Medical Publishing. This is the definitive work on medications and the breastfeeding mother. It is available for approximately $20 from Pharmasoft: 800-378-1317. Also, be sure to check Dr. Hale's Web site (address below)

Preston, J., and J. Johnson. 1997. *Clinical Psychopharmacology Made Ridiculously Simple.* 3rd ed. Miami: Medmaster. One of my personal favorites. This volume is written for physicians, but as the name implies, it concisely summarizes a wide range of information about antidepressants.

Raskin, V. 1997. *When Words Are Not Enough: The Women's Prescription for Depression and Anxiety.* New York: Broadway. A very thorough discussion of medications and side effects, written in a nurturing and helpful style.

American Psychological Association: 800-964-2000 or www.apa.org

Breastfeeding and Medication Information (Thomas Hale): www.neonatal.ttuhsc.edu/lact

Cognitive Therapy Referrals: www.feelinggood.com

National Mental Health Association: 800-969-NMHA or www.nmha.org

National Alliance for the Mentally Ill: 800-950-NAMI or www.nami.org

National Institute of Mental Health: 800-421-4211 or www.nimh.nih.gov

Resources for Natural Alternatives to Antidepressants

There is a great deal of information on alternatives to antidepressants, including all the options described throughout this chapter. All of these volumes are very helpful.

Balch, J. F., and P. A. Balch. 1997. *Prescription for Nutritional Healing,* 2nd ed. Garden City Park, N.Y.: Avery.

Bloomfield, H. H., M. Nordfors, and P. McWilliams. 1996. *Hypericum and Depression*. Los Angeles: Prelude.

Burns, D. D. 1999. *Feeling Good: The New Mood Therapy*. New York: Avon.

Cass, H. 1997. *St. John's Wort: Nature's Blues Buster*. Garden City Park, N.Y.: Avery.

Murray, M. T. 1996. *Natural Alternatives to Prozac*. New York: William Morrow & Co.

Nelson, M., with S. Wernick. 1998. *Strong Women Stay Young*. New York: Bantam.

Torkos, S., and K. A. Gazella. 1999. *Superior Healing Power of SAM-e*. Green Bay, Wis.: Impakt.

Wurtman, J. J., and S. Suffes. 1997. *The Serotonin Solution to Achieve Permanent Weight Control*. New York: Fawcett Columbine.

Another important source of information on herbs is the *German Commission E Monographs*. These are now available in English from the American Botanical Council at (512) 926-4900, www.herbalgram. org

American Herbal Pharmacopoeia: www.herbal-ahp.org
Herbs for Health magazine: subscribe at www.discoverherbs.com
National Center for Complementary and Alternative Medicine: www.nccam. nih.gov

CHAPTER 3

BURNOUT
WHEN YOU CAN'T GIVE ANY MORE

Are you drained? Do you wake up in the morning and wonder how you will get through the day? Are the people in your life exceptionally annoying? Are you withdrawing from others? Do you wonder whether anything you do really matters?

There comes a point when we can't give any more. If you are at that point, you may be suffering from mothering burnout. Burnout can be defined as a loss of enthusiasm, energy, idealism, perspective, and purpose; it has been described as trying to run a marathon at full speed. It is a state of total exhaustion—physical, mental, and spiritual—brought on by unrelenting stress. Burnout is a process during which a person disconnects from work and relationships. In the past twenty years, burnout has been noted in a wide variety of people-intensive professions, from teaching to nursing to police work.

Admitting that you are burned out doesn't mean you've failed. On the contrary, it's often the mothers who care the most who are the most prone to burnout. Pediatrician William Sears (1991) states mothers must be "on fire in order to be burned out" (195). In an article on the emotional strain of caring for an aging parent, psychologist Avrene Brandt (1998) makes a similar point:

> Those who are *most committed* and involved are most likely to become emotionally and physically exhausted. The myth that the harder you work and "the more you put in, the better it gets," does not work here. In fact, if you get hooked on this myth, you will neglect other important

aspects of your life, put your self-esteem at risk, and find yourself confronted with emotional reactions, which add to your stress.

It's not too late for you. Burnout is your mind and body's way of warning you that you need to make some changes. In this chapter, I'll describe some of the symptoms and stages of burnout, and the aspects of mothering that may make you vulnerable.

Common Signs of Burnout

A number of signs may indicate that you are burning out. You may experience any one of these or a combination of several (Potter 1998).

Negative Emotions

Everyone occasionally feels angry or sad. However, when anger or sadness becomes something you experience every day, it may be a sign of burnout. Another aspect of negative feelings is starting to doubt your ability to do what you're supposed to do: "If they knew the real me, they wouldn't think I was a good mother." You begin to feel like an imposter.

Some of these negative feelings could be related to unrealistic expectations you place on yourself about what a mother is supposed to be like. You may have the belief that mothers should give endlessly. You may also feel that you can't say "no" to anyone, especially your children. The inability to say "no" is remarkably common. *Working Mother* magazine found that only one-third of the mothers in a recent survey regularly set limits and boundaries with others. A full 54 percent indicated that they wanted to learn to say "no" when asked to take on an additional activity. (Cassidy 1999)

Interpersonal Problems

Problems with other people may also be an indication you are burning out. You may find yourself withdrawing, feeling frustrated with people, or overreacting to perceived misdeeds. You may become abrasive or harsh. Some of these behaviors may be a way to defend yourself against feelings of vulnerability or helplessness.

People in the helping professions who are burning out find themselves feeling cynical and insensitive to the needs of people in their care. You may find that you are increasingly impatient with your children or partner, and you may disengage or withdraw from the people you care about them.

Health Problems

As with stress and depression, burnout can bring a host of health problems. These include aches and pains, colds, headaches, inability to sleep, and chronic fatigue. By the end of the day, you may feel so worn out that all you can do is sit slack-jawed in front of the television. This happens to all of us once in a while. But when it gets to be a daily habit, take it as a warning. Exhaustion could also indicate the presence of depression or an underlying physical condition such as hypothyroidism. These possibilities should also be considered (see chapter 7).

Loss of Enthusiasm and Feelings of Meaningless

Burnout is often a time of existential crisis. You may find yourself questioning, perhaps for the first time, your role and the work you do. You may find you have lost interest in your work and your children. Everything seems like too much trouble. It may also seem that nothing you do matters. You may find yourself saying "Why bother?" or "Who cares?"

During this stage, your psychological defenses have worn down. Hurts and painful memories are starting to break through. You may find yourself overreacting to the smallest upset, and just feel miserable most of the time. You may even feel you don't know yourself anymore.

Substance Abuse and Unhealthy Behaviors

To cope with your feelings, you may find you are turning to alcohol or drugs. You may also find yourself eating too much, smoking too much, and drinking way too much coffee. All of these activities are physically depleting and compound the problem.

What Causes Burnout?

A variety of factors can put you at risk for burnout. Though many of these will also be described in upcoming chapters, here is a summary.

Unrealistic Expectations

Due to the cultural segregation of mothers and babies from the rest of life, many of you had very little experience with babies or small children before you became mothers. Suddenly, you're in charge of a small, helpless being. Because you haven't had lots of exposure and experience, you may underestimate the amount of work involved in child care. You may have adopted the naïve view that you can do it alone, not realizing how much you need a good support network.

Mothers internalize beliefs about what they should be and do. Often, these beliefs are unrealistic and even harmful, and they often take the form of "should" statements:

"A mother should anticipate all her family's needs"; "Mothers should be able to take care of everything"; "Mothers who take time off are lazy"; "Mothers should never get angry."

Cultural Messages

As children (and parents) of the information age, we are bombarded daily with hundreds of messages. At no other time in history has there been such an onslaught of images designed to sell products. In most families, mothers are the prime consumers, and most of these ads are directed at us. Advertisers try to make us feel bad about ourselves as women and as mothers. That is their goal. These messages are so pervasive that even when we see abundant evidence to the contrary, we believe the lies. Think about it: How many women do you know who have the flawless bodies you see in advertisements? How many families do you know who live in perfectly clean, impeccably decorated homes?

The power of image advertising is that we ourselves create the lie. If advertisers came out and *said* that if we bought their products, we'd have more friends, be more attractive, or be better mothers, we'd recognize it for the lie it is. But when they simply pair their products with symbols of the "good life," we create the lie and don't stop to analyze it.

Very high percentages of women are unhappy with their bodies. And we will often do things that are quite harmful to our health to meet the unrealistic ideal portrayed in advertisement and elsewhere. Barring that, we may feel secret shame that we are unable to meet such an ideal. Men don't do this. A very effective public service announcement has men sitting around complaining about their bodies. A blue-collar man sitting in a diner says: "I have my mother's thighs. I've always had my mother's thighs." You can imagine how ridiculous this sounds. And yet, if it was a group of women, we would probably think it was normal!

We also get quite a few messages about what mothers are supposed to do. Rarely on TV or in commercials do you see Cheerios on the floor, piles of unfolded laundry, big stacks of junk mail, or a bathroom that needs attention—unless it is an example of a really bad or incompetent mother. The documentary film *Killing Us Softly* highlights some of the more damaging examples in advertising—for instance a family that was very upset with a mother who made *too much cake.* This would not have been a problem in most families, I suspect. The ad was funny, but the message was clear—don't mess up or else your family will be mad at you. These advertisements try to create a "need" for their products. In order to do that, they make us feel bad.

Perfectionism

Perfectionism is a trap that many of us fall into. If you feel you have to do all things well, or that your best is never good enough, you are in danger of becoming burned out. I find that mothers who are survivors of childhood abuse are especially prone to perfectionism, especially in regard to their parenting. They try so hard to be good mothers that they feel they can't make *any* mistakes—that even their thoughts must always be loving and nurturing.

Perfectionism is often due to cognitive distortions described in chapter 2. The most common one is "all-or-nothing" thinking: that if I don't do everything perfectly, I'm a complete failure. Since no one can be perfect, a perfectionist may simply give up, disengaging from relationships and adopting a cynical, "what-difference-does-it-make?" attitude.

An Impossible Job

Unrealistic expectations are only part of the problem. Another part is that the job of mothering itself—if we do all that our culture implies is necessary—is truly impossible. Our culture sends some amazingly contradictory messages about what an ideal mother is like. Mothers try to live up to these ideals without recognizing the contradictions or the impossibility of the task. Like moths to the flame, you keep knocking yourselves out trying to do all the things our culture dictates.

As mothers, you are often expected to have a fulfilling career, time for personal interests, a rewarding marriage, involvement in your communities, a thorough grasp of current events—*and* be able to provide baked goods at a moment's notice. Your children should be attractive, smart, athletic, and well mannered. Your houses should be pretty and tastefully appointed, and of course, clean.

Below are some of the implied activities in the job of "mother." These are beyond the big responsibilities of child care and employment. Some of the activities in the list may be ones you enjoy. This listing doesn't mean you should cut activities you like. But I encourage you to consider whether you need to do them all, or do them all *now*, and also whether these activities are distributed fairly among members of your family. Are there things that others can do? (We'll revisit this topic in chapters 5 and 6.)

Meal Planning

As mothers, one of your functions is to plan for the sustenance of your families. Even if you don't do the actual cooking, quite frequently you are the ones who make the lists, buy the food, and coordinate the whole operation.

Home Decorating and Hospitality

You are often responsible for your surroundings—a job for which you may have little training. You are also responsible for opening your home to others and planning family events.

School Liaison

Mothers are frequently the ones who meet with teachers, chase after homework, make sure permission slips are signed, and bring cupcakes for birthdays. You may delegate these tasks, but often you are the ones who coordinate them. Mothers are the ones called if there is a problem at school. You make sure that school clothes and supplies are purchased, and that your children remember to bring something for "sharing." Or bring their lunch. Or bring their instrument to band practice.

Activity Coordination

In the movie *Baby Boom*, there is a scene where yuppie moms are flipping through thick Filofaxes trying to find a day when their kids can get together and play. Even at three and four years old, the kids in the movie are booked solid. While that depiction is obviously an exaggeration, for some families it is closer to reality than you might be comfortable admitting. There is scouting, soccer, and T-ball; there are lessons and church activities. No wonder many moms feel like they are always in the car.

Health and Safety

Who in your family makes the doctor and dentist appointments? Knows where the vaccination records are? Takes the kids for checkups? Remembers to schedule appointments before school starts? Who takes care of the animals? Or house plants? Or garden? While we're at it, who's responsible for taking the family pets to the vet? Whose job is it to keep the family supplied with toothpaste, toilet paper, and cold remedies? Who gets prescriptions filled? Who child-proofs your home? Who makes sure that fruits and vegetables get eaten? The health and safety of your families is in your hands.

Family Entertainment and Holidays

Who plans your family's outings? Or vacations? Or social engagements? Who buys or makes the Halloween costumes? Who cooks and coordinates the Thanksgiving feast? And let's talk Christmas! There are gifts, decorations, cards, and family pictures. Who makes sure everyone has appropriate matching outfits? And makes the date with the photographer? Several Jewish friends have told me that Hanukkah is getting similarly out of hand. And some families celebrate both holidays!

Relational Work

When there is an occasion to celebrate, who buys the gift? Who wraps and sends it? Who remembers the birthdays? Who sends the thank-you notes? Who buys the film, takes the pictures, gets them developed, and puts them in albums? Who keeps the family address book up to date?

The role of mother covers a very wide range of activities, many of which are never done. Mothers often feel that life is an endless treadmill. This brings us to the next cause of burnout: overwork.

41

Overwork

Remember the old expression: "A man works from sun to sun, but a woman's work is *never done*"? The futility of trying to finish work that is "never done" puts us at risk for burnout. Do you feel like all you do is work? Do you wish you could have a forty-eight-hour day? The sheer number of hours that mothers work during the day depletes the body. As you drag yourself through the day, struggling to meet your daily demands with a tired body, can mental and emotional fatigue be far behind? Work, both inside and outside the home, is such an important source of mothering stress that I have written the next three chapters about it.

Caregiving Overload

Like it or not, fair or not, in most families caregiving becomes the woman's responsibility. Caregiving can take many forms. You care for children, aging parents, and sick partners and friends. While caregiving can enrich you, it can also deplete you if you don't have support and take time for self-care.

Child Care

Even when employed outside the home, women do the bulk of the child care. And it is a source of contention in many relationships. This issue goes well beyond who changes diapers. It involves questions of daily care: Who feeds the children? Who stays home with a sick child? Who handles the nighttime routine? Who schleps to after-school activities? In some families, this type of child care is equitably divided, or the mother may do most of these activities by choice. In others, it is simply assumed that these are the mother's responsibilities (I'll discuss this more in chapter 6).

Children with Special Needs

Not all children are born equal. Some have special needs that may require more time and effort from you. Without help and support, you may be overwhelmed. Some children have "difficult" or "high-needs" temperaments. These are babies and children who seem to have an especially strong need to be with *you*. They don't separate well, want to be held a lot, and are almost superhuman in their lack of need for sleep. Even one child with a temperament like this can

CAN WE BLAME THE PROTESTANT WORK ETHIC?

Over the past few years, I've heard many people attribute our culture's workaholism to "the Protestant work ethic." This is interesting but not entirely accurate. The Puritans recommended that people work hard and not be idle ("Idle hands are the devil's workshop"). But there was an important difference between what they did and what we do. The Puritans, and members of other Christian sects, observed a weekly Sabbath, when they were prohibited (or strongly discouraged) from working. "Work" included cooking and all types of domestic work, hunting, fishing, boating, smoking or chewing tobacco, and using a horse, ox, or wagon if church was within walking distance. Men and women were expected to spend Sunday at church.

An informal Sabbath was observed for many years in this country even after we cut it from its religious moorings. Stores used to be closed on Sundays. Now we have the ability to work every day of the week. What would the Puritans think about our being able to work and shop twenty-four hours a day, seven days a week? And are we really better off for it?

send a mother into caregiving overload. The situation becomes more challenging when a mother has one or more children with a high-needs temperaments, and other children to care for as well.

Children may also have difficulties in school in the form of learning disabilities or attention-deficit hyperactivity disorder (ADHD). Parents may find they spend an extraordinary amount of time trying to secure services for their children or helping their children with schoolwork at night. To compound the difficulties, because they struggle in school these children may also develop some social characteristics that isolate them from peers or make them a target for bullies.

Babies or children with chronic illnesses can dramatically increase caregiving responsibilities. Of course, the amount of caregiving varies considerably depending on the condition the child has. But caring for a child with health concerns takes time and may overwhelm you, bringing you at times to "a state beyond fatigue that is akin to despair" (Greenspan 1998, 42). This is especially true if you have other children at home in addition to your child with health issues. You may feel isolated because it is difficult for others to understand what you are going through (see chapters 9 and 10).

Closely Spaced Children and Multiples

Having children closely spaced in age can also lead to caregiving overload, since the caregiving tasks are unrelenting. These caregiving responsibilities may be so intense in the early days that everything else goes on hold: the house, the job, friends. According to Karen Gromada, author of *Mothering Multiples* (1999), mothers can get so task focused that they stop thinking of their children as children. Days may disappear into a blur of feeding and diapering, feeding and diapering. And it's easy to lose yourself in this routine, as Suzanne, a mother of twin infants, describes:

> I'm TOTALLY overwhelmed by these two tiny creatures. Are you people all superhuman, or wealthy enough to afford armies of help? How, oh how, do you take care of infant twins by yourself? When they are both crying at the same time, and there's no one else there to pick up one while I pick up the other one, and I am completely sleep deprived, WHAT AM I SUPPOSED TO DO???

When there are several small children in your home to care for, you have no downtime. Sleep deprivation is a particular problem. Sometimes mothers are just overwhelmed by the sheer amount of work involved in baby or child care.

Stress and arguing increase when families have multiples, as this parent describes:

> We've . . . been married for six years, but the last three with the kids have added a depth and craziness I could have never imagined. Sometimes I see a bit too clearly how parents of multiples can get divorced, so it was nice to hear I'm not alone in struggling. I can tell you that being parents of multiples is about the hardest thing on a marriage that I know of.

Chores and taking care of the children are two big sources of arguments. Often, both parents are working so hard and sleeping so little that they snap at each other. Only the most crucial chores get done in the first few months, but other projects start piling up around the house. When families have more than one small child at home, in order to survive, they need to let go of some of the standards of cleanliness they had before the kids were born.

Another factor complicating the picture for many mothers of multiples, in particular, is that their pregnancy or adoption may have come about after years of infertility treatment. If you adopted your babies, you may also find yourself feeling isolated from other mothers of multiples simply due to the differences in your experiences. In either case, these are babies you really wanted, so how can you complain? This kind of thinking may not allow you to acknowledge the real difficulties associated with a multiple birth or adoption. The support of others in the same boat can help as this mother discovered:

> I went to my first Mothers of Twins meeting when I was five months pregnant. I didn't feel that I belonged at all. It seemed that everyone was there to complain about how difficult it was to raise twins or triplets. I believed I would be able to become a parent to my twins without voicing a single complaint, frustration, or negative feeling. After all, I put my whole being into trying to become a parent—how could I possibly find anything less than perfect about the experience? Now that I have lived the overwhelming exhaustion of the early months as every parent of multiples does and dealt with the day-to-day logistical issues, I join into these frustration-venting conversations among parents of multiples without a second thought.

Single Parenting

According to the U.S. Census Bureau, there are 10 million single mothers in the United States, up 133 percent since 1970 (Bryson and Casper 1998). Single parents often tell me that they did not know the meaning of stress until they started to parent on their own. Single parents also report having no downtime from relentless child-care activities. Loneliness and isolation can also be particular challenges for the single mother. And as I described in chapter 2, mother-headed households also have a higher likelihood of poverty.

These issues are somewhat easier to face if you are a single parent by choice, though the challenges are still very real. But if you are single against your will either through death or divorce, the issues of single parenting more commonly lead to anger, depression, and burnout. Devon and Elizabeth's husbands left them for other women. Both of them had three young children to raise alone with little or no child support. Devon had to struggle with depression. She had so little money that she sometimes wondered how she would make it through the day. She didn't want to put her children in day care. So she decided to do day care in her home instead. Money was always a problem, and she subsisted for several years just above the poverty level. Elizabeth also felt depressed and overwhelmed. She found it difficult to care for her children. Some days, their needs were too much for her. She was also very angry: angry at her husband, angry at friends of her husband who seemed unable to make him stay, angry at other women whose husbands had not left them, and angry at God for allowing this to happen to her.

Whether your partner left or died, you may feel all the kinds of anger Elizabeth did, and more. Unfortunately, you may also feel the urge to take this anger out on your children. It is especially important that you seek support and find ways to express your anger in healthy ways. Some examples of this are writing in a journal, speaking to a therapist, or joining a support group.

Anne, a single mother of two teens, describes the total exhaustion that comes with caring for her children, one of whom has special needs, and having no time for herself. Even before her divorce, she felt totally overwhelmed by her life. After a long illness, she took her kids to visit her parents. She describes this period as "one of the low points of my life":

> As I lay in bed at my parents' house, I experienced the horrible longing that death would overtake me and my son. I was feeling completely suffocated by my husband and kids. I had nothing else to give them, and was getting nothing in return. I was sure that if my son and I were not in anyone's lives, everyone would be better off. I had birthed, breastfed, and cared for my two children for almost six years at this point. I was home-schooling them as well.

> Six years and a divorce later, I learned that my son has a form of autism. No wonder I was struggling! Knowing this has changed many aspects of my life. Though he receives help now, my life has been permanently altered and complicated by his condition. As a single parent, I have had to persevere through the trials of getting my son the education he needs, facing the fallout of the teasing and harrassment he receives, working full-time at a low-paying job, putting my own career goals on hold, juggling the needs of two very different and high-need children, and finding stolen moments for myself.

> I have virtually no social life. I have very little time alone. I am facing the challenges of raising two teenagers at this point. Through all the grieving and loss of dreams, I have

learned that we are indeed spiritual beings having a human experience. Each day I need to rediscover this or I simply cannot cope. In the end I want to know that I have, in good conscience, done the best I knew how at the time.

Aging Parents

As our population ages, more women will find themselves caring for aging parents. Nearly one in four families is currently providing care for an elderly family member or friend, a number that is expected to increase (U.S. Department of Labor 1998). Family members are the people most likely to provide this care, with 41 percent of care providers being adult children (National Academy on an Aging Society 2000). According to the U.S. Department of Labor, 72 percent of caregivers are women, and women provide the majority of care for aging relatives. For example, women spent an average of 19.9 hours per week in direct and indirect care compared to the 11.8 hours spent by men (U.S. Department of Labor 1998).

Women between the ages of thirty and fifty are often called the "sandwich generation," in that they must often provide care for both children and parents. Approximately 41 percent of women caring for elderly relatives are also caring for children under age eighteen. The Department of Labor put together a profile of the typical caregiver. She is a forty-six-year-old woman who is employed and also spends around eighteen hours per week caring for her mother who lives nearby. The number of hours is even higher in some families. Approximately 1.5 million families spend twenty to forty hours a week caring for an elderly family member, and another 4 million spend at least 40 hours a week. The study also found that elder caregiving has an impact on work, causing caregivers to come in late, work fewer hours, and even give up work or retire early.

In some cases, providing care for aging parents is voluntary. In other cases, there is no real choice. The amount of work also varies tremendously. Is the parent nearby? Is she living with your family? What is the degree of her impairment? Sometimes people who are chronically ill can become very depressed, or have badly impaired cognitive function, making them need that much more care. For example, Mary's father became increasingly verbally abusive each time she spoke with him. Rhonda's mother, on the other hand, became more physically frail each year, requiring more and more assistance on a daily basis.

The difficulty of caring for an aging relative is compounded when you don't feel you had a choice in the matter. Anger and resentment are common. If your parent was abusive or neglectful

47

while you were growing up, you might be very angry at having to care for this parent now. The phenomenon of elder abuse and neglect demonstrates that caregivers can get overwhelmed and react in destructive ways.

"Codependency" and Overinvolvement

Codependency is a word that has been so overused, it is almost a cliché. Nevertheless, it's often the women who take on everyone else's troubles who are at highest risk for burning out. There is nothing wrong with being concerned about and caring for other people, but carrying their problems may overwhelm us. You need your wisdom when trying to determine how to spend your limited time, and fortitude in putting some limits on how involved you get in problems that are not your own.

Often, the tendency to cross a line of involvement is based in your family of origin. In one recent study, women with chronic stressors in their families of origin such as childhood abuse, parental addiction, or parental illness were more likely to be codependent (Fuller and Warner 2000). Sometimes, too, a significant loss or traumatic event in adulthood can lead to an overinvolvement in the problems of others. Lynn's story reflects some of the strain that too many outside commitments can create. Some of these difficulties she relates to her son's death.

> I am a fifty-two-year old wife and mother of two daughters. I lost a son to SIDS fourteen years ago. My volunteer work includes working with breastfeeding mothers and treasurer at the county level of a political party. I work four hours a day as a receptionist in a civil engineering office. I have had breast cancer twice.

Lynn took a helping call from a breastfeeding mother whose baby was not gaining weight. After researching the situation, she realized that the baby might die.

> That night I couldn't sleep. I was inconsolable. I could not stop crying or thinking about this baby. In the morning I called the mother back and told her how worried I was, and that her baby needed supplements immediately.

Her worry continued through another night of no sleep and crying. She recognized that she needed to turn this situation over to someone else.

It became apparent that I was burning out. I made frantic phone calls trying to find someone who would take care of this mother. I did find relief. I mailed a packet of information to the mother and was in bed for three days after that.

I believe this situation tapped into my unresolved grief about my son's SIDS death as an infant. The stress of the past month crashed down on me as I let go of my control and cried. But I couldn't turn off the tears, and that was the sign that I was over the top. I have been exhausted since, but functioning. I know I need to let go of some things but I value all these aspects of my life highly!

What You Can Do

You have probably noticed that many of the symptoms of burnout are similar to those of depression. One aspect of burnout can be chronic depression. Depending on how bad your symptoms are, you may need to seek the assistance of a mental health professional. But there are also a number of steps you can take. Burnout is something you should pay attention to. The good news is that you don't have to go through your life in misery.

Stop Denying

When you are burned out, you often don't recognize it. If you are dragging yourself through each day, admit it and resolve to take some positive action. Acknowledge the stresses and pressures in your life, and start paying attention to all the stress-related symptoms you are probably feeling. It's time to make some changes.

Get Reconnected

People have a natural tendency to withdraw from others when they are under stress. Burnout compounds this by making us irritable and impatient. If you are laboring under perfectionism, you might also withdraw from others for fear that they will discover that you are not perfect, or because you are annoyed by their imperfections.

When you are burned out, one of the first things you need to do is reconnect with others. Start with your family. Set aside time to be with your partner and children. This is also time to get together with some of the friends you maybe haven't seen for a while. It's important that you reconnect with people who can give back to you.

You might also consider some volunteer work. That may seem a strange suggestion if you are already overwhelmed. And it may not be for everyone. But sometimes being involved in the lives of others can expand your perspective beyond your own problems. Caution: If you tend toward getting *too* involved in people's problems, be careful not to take on too much.

Set Some Boundaries

You may find that you have been taking on too much in several areas of your life. Are you the one people always come to with their problems? Do you try to do everything yourself? Do you have trouble saying "no"? You must learn to set some limits. You are, after all, only human. Stop trying to meet everyone's needs. Does this mean that you should stop caring about others? Of course not! But you can put some reasonable limits on how you handle their requests. If friends always want to talk about their problems, but never yours, perhaps you can limit the frequency with which this occurs by not always being available to discuss their problems in depth. Or set a time limit on these conversations. You might find that this is better for them too. When a request to do something comes in, realistically evaluate whether it will be possible for you at that time. Say "no" occasionally. If you freely choose to do something, it will be much more enjoyable than if you feel coerced. If you need some help with saying no, as many women do, check out Henry Cloud and John Townsend's book *Boundaries* (1992).

Get Some Help with Your Work

When you are faced with too much work, try to do less of it. For jobs that you decide must be done, start delegating as much as you can. You are not the only one who can do most types of work. Can you get a teenager to give you a hand in the afternoon? Can you swap baby-sitting with another mother? Think creatively.

This gets tricky when you are a caregiver. Sometimes it really does need to be you. However, there may be some type of respite care available, including adult day care centers and visiting nurses for aging parents. And don't forget the others living under your roof. All except the youngest children can pick up after themselves and help put stuff away, and this goes for your partner as well. It is essential that you stop trying to do it all yourself (we'll revisit this topic again in chapter 6).

Get Treatment for Depression

Depression can be a significant part of your burnout. If you think that you might be depressed, look into your treatment options (see chapter 2) and take care of it.

Stop Mentally Rehearsing Your Daily Difficulties

As I've mentioned in previous chapters, you need to pay attention to negative self-talk. When you are in a burned-out phase of life, you can make matters worse by going through the day thinking "my life stinks." It may, at the moment. But constantly thinking this does not help you at all. Instead, try to think creatively about how you can change the situation.

Some Final Thoughts

Burnout may feel hopeless to you. Fortunately, it is not. Keep reading. Many of the chapters that follow will more specifically address concerns and problems that are making you feel bad. There is a light at the end of this tunnel.

For Further Reading

There have been a number of good books written about burnout. Here are a few of my favorites. They provide a good overview of burnout and offer a number of helpful suggestions.

Books on Burnout

Minirth, F., et al. 1997. *Beating Burnout: Balanced Living for Busy People.* New York: Inspirational Press.

Potter, B. 1998. *Overcoming Job Burnout: How to Renew Enthusiasm for Work.* Berkeley, Calif.: Ronin.

Reinhold, B. B. 1997. *Toxic Work: How to Overcome Stress, Overload, and Burnout, and Revitalize Your Career.* New York: Plume.

Books on Perfectionism

These are two of the best books for dealing with perfectionism. They are written on depression, but both address the faulty cognitions that underlie perfectionism. In *Feeling Good*, there are chapters on perfectionism and approval addiction, challenging readers to "dare to be average."

Burns, D. 1999. *Feeling Good: The New Mood Therapy*. New York: Avon. See especially Chapters 10–14.

Burns, D. 1999. *The Feeling Good Handbook*. New York: Plume. See Chapters 9–10.

Resources for Caregiving Overload

Card, E., with C. Watts Kelly. 1996. *The Single Parent's Money Guide*. New York: Macmillan Spectrum.

Gromada, K. 1999. *Mothering Multiples*. Schaumburg, Ill.: La Leche League International.

Nelsen, J., C. Erwin, and C. Delzer. 1994. *Positive Discipline for Single Parents: A Practical Guide to Raising Children Who Are Responsible, Respectful, and Resourceful*. Rocklin, Calif.: Prima Publishing.

Noel, J. B., with A. Klein. 1998. *The Single Parent Resource*. Beverly Hills, Calif.: Champion Press.

Weishett, E. 1994. *Aging Parents: When Mom and Dad Can't Live Alone Anymore*. Elgin, Ill.: Lion Publishing.

Web Sites for Single Mothers

M.O.M.S.: Single Moms on a Mission: www.singlemoms.org
Parents Without Partners: www.parentswithoutpartners.org
Single Parents Association: www.singleparents.org

Web Sites for Mothers of Multiples

Mothers of Supertwins (MOST): www.mostonline.org
National Organization of Mothers of Twins Clubs: www.nomotc.org
Triplet Connection: www.tripletconnection.org

Resources for Elder Care

Aging Network Services: 301-657-4329 or www.agingnets.com
American Association of Retired Persons: 202-434-2277 or www.aarp.com
Children of Aging Parents (CAPS): 800-227-7294 or www.careguide.com/careguide.cgi/caps/capshome.htm!
ElderCare Online: www.ec-online.net

CHAPTER 4

HEARTH AND HOME
THE FASCINATING HISTORY OF WOMEN'S DOMESTIC WORK IN AMERICA

Mothers are bombarded with advice and cultural messages about how to clean our houses, raise our children, and spend our days. No matter what we do, many of us have a vague sense of guilt about not "doing enough."

If you find yourself feeling guilty without really understanding why, read on. There are historical and cultural forces that you may not be aware of that are probably shaping your beliefs about who you are and what you should be accomplishing. Ruth Schwartz Cowan, in her history of household technology (1983), describes the influence of these cultural forces this way:

> Many of the rules that tyrannize housewives are unconscious and therefore potent. By exploring their history we can bring these rules into consciousness and thereby dilute their potency. . . . If we can learn to select among the rules only those that make sense for us in the present, we can begin to control household technology instead of letting it control us. (219)

History can be wonderfully informative, giving a perspective that few other things can. And history is a common reference point. Conservatives and liberals alike refer to the "traditional family." Usually, this means the family structure of the 1950s. But as you'll see, in order to understand where we are now, we need to go back further than fifty years. Indeed, the traditional family, as it's currently conceptualized, has its origins in the period of time before the Civil War, the Antebellum period.

In this chapter, I provide a brief history of women's work both inside and outside the home over the last 175 years or so. I've used three primary historical texts: *Domestic Revolutions: A Social History of American Family Life* (Mintz and Kellogg 1988), *More Work for Mother* (Schwartz Cowan 1983), and *"Just a Housewife": The Rise and Fall of Domesticity in America* (Matthews 1987). Inevitably, my discussion will have some limitations. Within any of the eras I cover, there have of course been mothers who were able to carve out for themselves satisfying lives even when it seemed that the broader culture was against them. Further, there are vast differences in the experiences of mothers based not only on when they lived, but their social class and ethnic heritage. Finally, I want to acknowledge that even when a culture did support mothers, there were women who felt confined by their role and were unhappy. Culture alone cannot govern relationships that occur in individual families, but I hope this information will help you recognize the cultural forces that shape your own life.

Women of the Antebellum Period

From 1830 to 1860, the status of the American housewife was at its peak. Historian Glenna Matthews outlines several reasons for this. In the years following the Revolutionary War, "home" began to become a place of emotional attachment, a haven in a harsh world, where children and adults were nurtured. These changes represented a fundamental cultural shift. Prior to the Revolutionary War, fathers were considered responsible for raising children. In custody disputes, with few exceptions, fathers were granted custody. The few parenting

It is the correct thing to remember that the lady who rules the household must have absolute authority in it and rule as absolute queen. No comfort or order can be obtained without this . . . The lady who holds this position must remember that the every-day happiness of those in the home circle is in her hands; that she has the greatest power of anyone to make the home a place of peace and happiness, or a place to avoid. (from M.C., *Everybody's Book of Correct Conduct, Being the Etiquette of Every-day Life,* 1893) books that existed during this time were addressed to fathers. It was many years before mothers were considered better nurturers of children "of tender years."

With the rise in the status of the home, the role of the mother was elevated. In a young country, embarking on "the grand experiment" of democracy, mothers came to be seen as the moral center of the culture. There was much emphasis on mothers being the trainers of the citizenry. As such, they needed to be educated and thoroughly knowledgeable about the issues and concerns of the day. For the first time, the literacy rate of boys and girls was about equal (Matthews 1987).

Domesticity had a high place in the broader culture. The "notable housewife" was a frequent theme in fiction, and she was positively portrayed. Her role required a great deal of skill. Female craft traditions such as cooking, baking, and stitchery became jealously guarded family treasures that were passed from mother to daughter.

This is not to romanticize the work of mothers during this time. Much of the work in housewifery was grueling and unrelenting. There were limited opportunities for women. Women could not vote, and married women could not own property. Looking at the lives of these women through modern eyes, we would note that their work was largely segregated by sex and limited to the domestic realm. Some individual women wrote in letters and journals that they were overwhelmed with the responsibilities of child care and running a household.

As difficult as it was, however, women's domestic work was infused with transcendent meaning that came from both religious and secular sources. Although aspects of their work were hard and tedious, they were constantly told that they were making a significant contribution to their country. Women of the antebellum period were raising citizens for the new republic. The importance of this role was extolled from the pulpits. According to Matthews (1987) there was a turning from the more rigid Calvinism of the Puritans to an emphasis on God's grace. This influenced how children were treated within the home. Mothers and fathers were supposed to be living examples to their children of God's love.

Many of the ideas about the notable housewife may, in fact, have come from the Bible. In the Old Testament book of Proverbs, we see an example of a notable housewife in "the virtuous woman" of Chapter 31 (verses 10 to 31). Her primary sphere is domestic, yet she has interest in the wider world. She works hard; is competent; handles money; buys and sells land; manufactures goods for herself, her family, and to sell; provides for her family; and helps the poor and needy. Her husband has status in the community because of her efforts. Both her husband and children praise her and "call her blessed."

Secular support of the notable housewife came from nineteenth-century philosophers such as Ralph Waldo Emerson, one of the most important intellectuals of his time. Domestic themes were also present in the works of Nathaniel Hawthorne. For both Hawthorne and Emerson, the model American home was loving, welcoming for visitors, free of social caste, and inhabited by a family that could be emulated.

The importance of mothers and other domestic themes were also key in the growing movements for the abolition of slavery and for women's suffrage. As Matthews (1987) states: ". . . the domestic sphere was not viewed as an ahistorical enclave where people could meet basic needs . . . but rather as a dynamic scene of actions that could affect the outcome of history" (57). Women reformers used the moral authority of the home to highlight the plight of the less fortunate. One of the most famous exemplars of this is Harriet Beecher Stowe. We all know her as the author of the remarkable *Uncle Tom's Cabin*, a book that Abraham Lincoln credited as ultimately bringing about the end of slavery. The book also prominently presents themes of home and motherhood.

Shortly after the death of her infant son Charley she wrote *Uncle Tom's Cabin*—the first book that addressed the issue of slavery. Her experience of mourning a child gave her empathy for the slave mother who could lose her children by having them sold away from her. Eliza, one of her main characters, is a slave who runs away with her young son to keep him from being sold.

In *Uncle Tom's Cabin*, the homes of the characters are also very much evidence of their moral stature. The home of the Quaker couple who offers refuge to Eliza is cheerful, neat, and warm—the embodiment of Beecher Stowe's most deeply held beliefs. In contrast, the home of the villainous Simon Legree is filthy, ragged, and slovenly. But merely keeping house well was not enough; notable housewives needed to be of good character as well. An example here is the character of the cousin who comes to take over the household. She handles her duties well, but it is not until she overcomes her prejudice that she is granted notable housewife status.

The importance of women's being knowledgeable citizens and using their influence for good was something Beecher Stowe believed throughout her life. However, the perception of women's role in the broader culture would undergo a change after the Civil War.

The Decline of Domesticity: 1865 to 1920

The decline of domesticity began in the years after the Civil War, which ended in 1865. The notable housewife was no longer a theme in literature. Rather, she was gradually replaced with the overbearing mother, or "housewife bitch," who soon became prominent in literature. Matthews (1987) cites numerous examples from the writings of Sinclair Lewis and George Peck, author of the *Peck's Bad Boy* series. No longer the moral center of the family and the culture, mothers were seen as the problem.

Matthews hypothesizes that these negative images of housewives started to appear because of the perception that the housewife/activist had in fact gained too much power. Many women's groups, such as the powerful Women's Christian Temperance Union (WCTU), used their activism to try to curb traditionally male behaviors such as drinking and gambling. A backlash was perhaps inevitable: "Politicizing the home and then turning this to female advantage inevitably made enemies for domestic values, enemies who would welcome a diminution in the sanctity of home" (Matthews 1987, 91).

But negative portrayals in literature of housewives were only the beginning of change in how mothers were perceived. Soon, industrialization and modern science would also change the role of the housewife, and change it forever.

Industrialization, Consumerism, and Women's Work: 1920 to 1960

Several cultural forces severely eroded the status of the American housewife during the early and mid-twentieth century. Certainly one of the most pervasive was industrialization, which started about 1860. One of its first changes in the household was that it created an even more marked division of labor between the sexes than had existed previously, as men left the home to go to work in offices and factories. And its influence did not stop there.

The Laborsaving Device

Industrialization also had a large influence on women's work with the invention of the laborsaving device. Such devices—washing machines, sewing machines, and vacuum cleaners—were designed to make the onerous tasks of taking care of a home less burdensome. They were also designed to eliminate the need for servants. These intentions were not bad, but the devices had unforeseen long-term effects on the work women did.

First, laborsaving devices clearly did make some tasks easier, but they simultaneously raised the standards. For example, since cleaning now took less time, the yardstick of "cleanliness" rose. Since it was easier to wash clothing with a washing machine, women could now wash clothes more often. As family diets became more varied, cooking became more complex. Larger homes meant more to clean. Finally, work that had traditionally been hired out (at least in middle-class homes) returned home and became the job of the housewife. These tasks included laundry, rug and drapery cleaning, and floor polishing (Schwartz Cowan 1983).

Before the advent of laborsaving devices, most middle-class homes had at least some domestic help. With the machines, women did most of these chores alone. Indeed, Schwartz Cowan describes how the housewife of the 1950s could single-handedly produce what her counterpart in the 1850s needed a staff of three or four to produce: middle-class standards of health and cleanliness for her family. Laborsaving devices eliminated much drudgery but not the labor or time needed for household tasks: even with the new products and machines, women were still working the same number of hours as women in previous generations. "There was more work for a mother to do in a modern home because there was no one left to help her with it" (Schwartz Cowan 1983, 201).

Laborsaving devices also had other insidious effects. Since the technology was "new," kitchens and households were now redesigned to accommodate these machines. Women had to rely on outside experts rather than their mothers or each other to help them use, manage, and repair the new technology. What had traditionally been their sphere of expertise suddenly became foreign.

Finally many tasks that required skill were eliminated. In fact, time management experts told women to make their household tasks as automatic and "brainless" as possible. The problem no one had foreseen was that housework "continued to fill women's time while it starved their brains" (Matthews 1987, 195). The malaise of the housewife was first identified in 1920 by Dr. Abraham Myerson, in a book entitled *The Nervous Housewife*. He also identified isolation as a particular problem for the housewife, as were the deskilling and devaluation of her job. In 1930, in *Ladies' Home Journal*, he added one more problem to the list: the devaluation of motherhood itself (cited in Matthews, 1987).

The Army of Experts

Knowledge that was traditionally transmitted woman to woman began to be considered obsolete. We now needed to be taught by "experts" how to cook, raise our children, and run our households. Immigrant families were told to shed their traditions in favor of "modern" techniques. When groups resisted and continued to practice their old ways, they were often objects of derision and pity. In this way, the dominant white, middle-class culture attempted to force its views on women of other cultures—often with success.

During this time, home economists such as Charlotte Perkins Gilman became exasperated with the inefficiency of the American housewife. She argued that women must be freed from domestic work so that they could do "more important" things. She proposed community kitchens, where all families in a community could eat together; communal child rearing; and provision of outside services, such as laundry, for the family. She believed that housework should be done by professionals instead of "amateurs" at home. Economist Juliet Schor (1992) describes Gilman's proposed solutions in positive terms, making the broader point that the reason most homes and home appliances are not designed with ease of care in mind is that we don't value women's time. That may be true. But we should be careful not to adopt our culture's negative attitude about women or domestic work which is evident when we speak of housewives' "inefficiency" or the "unimportance" of their work.

As more items were mass-produced, fewer were created at home. Women were no longer responsible for making cloth or clothing, soap or candles. And clearly, many women (if not most) relished being released from these tasks. Yet something was lost when women's domestic work was deskilled. Women in the past had concrete evidence of their productivity and contribution to the family. They could point to vegetables grown, jars of preserves put up, clothing sewn, cloth woven. Many of these household tasks were also outlets for women's creativity.

Sewing, quilting, lace-making, stitchery, and some kinds of cooking became dramatically less common during the twentieth century as mass-produced items came to be considered better than what women could produce themselves. Many of the daily tasks women now performed lacked any kind of permanency. Cleaning, diapering, and driving were all tasks that had to be done over and over, and there was often no evidence that they had ever been done at all. In *Motherhood Stress* (1989), Debbie Lewis describes this lack of permanent products and speculates that this is why so many at-home mothers enjoy various types of needlework: they know the product they create will last for more than five minutes.

Scientific Eating

With tremendous arrogance, home economists and other experts told women that they could no longer rely on the palates of their families to tell them what food was "good." Instead, women needed to rely on nutritionists to tell them what their families should eat. "Scientifically engineered" food substitutes began finding their way into American homes. These were widely touted in women's magazines, which described those who resisted as ridiculous when they failed to embrace the modern way. Interestingly, the native cuisines of many immigrant families were not so easy to change. These families ignored the pitch for scientifically engineered foods and continued to eat their traditional diets.

Commercially baked bread did not catch on until the early 1900s, and other substitutes for homemade food did not really catch on until there were food shortages during World War II. Curiously, after the war, these foods were marketed as "better" than the foods they were designed to replace. Canned, packaged, and mass-marketed foods eventually took over the market, and have become so much the norm that foods prepared from fresh ingredients taste strange, especially to kids. Matthews (1987) describes her dismay at this development:

> Arguably, the nadir of American cookery came in the fifties. This was the heyday of prepared foods and the cream-of-mushroom-soup cuisine whereby the cook could pour a can of this product over anything that was not dessert and create a culinary treat according to the standards of the day. (211)

Cream-of-mushroom cuisine appears to be making a comeback as advertisers capitalize on baby boomers' nostalgia for their youth.

We are still reaping the consequences of the marketing campaigns that brought scientifically engineered foods into our homes. Consider the campaign to promote margarine as being healthier than butter. Now we have learned that trans fatty acids (which are in both margarine and most commercial baked goods) are as bad, or even worse for you than the saturated fat and cholesterol in butter. I wonder if the chemically laden fat-free products now flooding the market will have a similar history. We're eating more and more of these foods and finding ourselves, as a country, fatter than ever. A growing body of research evidence indicates there is a connection.

As with other forms of fake food, breastmilk substitutes appeared on the scene in the 1920s. These substitutes were called "formula" in reference to their scientific origin. Formula was marketed for decades as being *better* for the health of babies. Studies from that era demonstrated the tragic error of this claim; for instance, one study found that babies who were fed formula had a mortality rate that was three to six times higher than babies who were breastfed (Woodbury 1925). Eighty years later, hundreds of scientific studies have confirmed the inferiority of this scientifically engineered product.

Scientific Mothering

A parallel development occurred with regard to child rearing. Rather than feeding babies when they appeared hungry, women were no longer to trust these cues. Instead they were to rely on outside experts to determine when and how often babies should eat. This approach had a disastrous impact on breastfeeding. When feedings are rigidly scheduled, a mother's milk supply decreases. But that was okay according to the experts of the day, since bottle-feeding allowed a much more scientific approach. Intake could now be accurately measured. Unfortunately, variations of this approach still exist today.

According to psychologists such as John B. Watson, parents were to mold children's behavior through a process of positive and negative reinforcements. In fact, Watson openly questioned whether mothers were the best ones to be raising children, given their lack of a scientific education. (I often wonder if John Watson knew any actual children.)

> It is a serious question in my mind whether children should know their parents. There are undoubtedly much more scientific ways of bringing up children, which will probably mean finer and happier children. (Cited in Matthews 1987, 183)

His comments have an eerily modern ring to them. In a 1997 book about overbearing social welfare policies and their negative effects on families, Dana Mack observes:

> Our family policy, it seems, has been based upon a long-standing conviction on the part of educators, psychol-

ogists, and social service professionals that parents really should not be too heavily engaged in the child-rearing process, but rather should abandon it to professionals. (21)

Mothers of the twentieth century were warned that they must abandon the child-rearing techniques of previous generations, whereby mothers kissed and coddled their young children. Parents were advised to let their babies cry. They were told to adopt a strict regimen for feeding, sleeping, and toileting so that they conditioned a child to be polite and cleanly. Mothers were told that they could start bowel training at age one month by inserting a tapered soap stick into the rectum for three to five minutes (Mintz and Kellogg 1988). Much of this child-rearing advice now seems ridiculous, if not cruel.

Other female traditions, such as herbal medicine and midwifery, were also all but lost as conventional (read: "scientific") medicine began to take hold. More traditional forms of healing were relegated to the category of "old wives' tales" and dismissed out of hand. These other forms of healing were quite prominent in the nineteenth century and earlier, only to almost die out in the first sixty or seventy years of the twentieth . We are now only beginning to realize what we lost by the abandonment of all these traditions. And while alternative (read: traditional) medicine has become increasingly popular, there is still strong opposition to it from segments of the scientific community.

Consumerism

Industrialization brought us another aspect of modern life: consumerism. By the 1920s, large numbers of mass-produced consumer goods were within the financial reach of the average family. In order to create a market for these items, the advertising industry was born. With it came the marketing of obsolescence and "creative waste." The idea was to train women to buy new items rather than use everything to the very end: in a telling phrase, in Christine Fredrick's 1929 volume *Selling to Mrs. Consumer*, to "waste more rather than less" (cited in Matthews 1987, 170). Consumerism has as its foundation the chronic "need" to purchase new goods without considering whether the item is really needed, whether it's durable, or how it was produced. Consumerism is a trend that continues to strengthen to this day, and whose impact is felt not only in our overflowing homes, but on our overflowing planet.

As we discussed in chapter 3, advertising also erodes women's self-esteem. Mothers were (and are) repeatedly told that if their families were not healthy, attractive, and popular, and if they themselves were haggard-looking or tired, it was *their fault,* since the means to remedy these problems were easily available. Guilt continues to be one of the most common appeals used in advertising to women (Schwartz Cowan 1983).

Industrialization and the growth of consumer culture also had an impact on community life in general. As more and more products became available for purchase, the value of neighbor helping neighbor began to fade. In a work published in 1898, Alice Morse Earle spoke of the decline in community:

> We nowadays have generalized our sentiments; we have more philanthropy and less neighborliness; we have more love for mankind and less for men. We are independent of our neighbors, but infinitely more dependent on the world at large. The personal element has been removed to a large extent from our social ethics. We buy nursing and catering just as we hire our houses built and buy our corn ready ground. Doubtless everything we buy is infinitely better; nevertheless, our loss in affectionate zeal is great. (390)

No doubt, purchasing services from professionals rather than having them come via relationships would appeal to many who opted for the scientific approach. But others realized that a great deal was also lost.

The Automobile

Another impact of industrialization was the advent and increasing availability of the automobile. As early as 1925, it was in widespread use. The car became the means by which the American housewife did most of her work, and where she spent most of her time (Schwartz Cowan 1983). Mothers spent a large part of their day chauffeuring other members of the family, a situation that has not improved. But there were problems associated with the car being women's primary place of work. First, by the end of the day, they could not point to something tangible that they had accomplished. Second, driving also had the effect of isolating women from each other. Rather than having a place where they could gather, they were encased in their individual automobiles.

The Low Status of Housewives

The popular literature of the day also continued to attack American housewives in several ways. Some plays, novels, and films presented the idea of "home" being a place of emotional attachment as a joke and women at home were portrayed as idle, or even as parasites. At the same time, women's magazines and advertisements advised women to create a haven for their husbands at home. But unlike their counterparts of 100 years earlier, creating this haven entailed being deliberately "dumb" about the goings-on in the outside world. During the 1930s and 1940s, the *Ladies' Home Journal* repeatedly told women not to be concerned or involved in the world outside their homes. In an article published in September 1938, Bruce and Beatrice Gould issued the following advice:

> Be glad you're dumb about all these earth-shaking questions. They don't affect you nearly so much as a lot of other things much nearer home. . . . The great problems of the world are all Greek to you—but the problems of your home and family and community are right down your alley. Be glad you're dumb while your husband is saving the world—be brave and you can save the home. (Cited in Matthews 1987, 198)

Contrast this with the mother who was responsible for the education of citizens of the new republic 100 years previously.

While the technological advances of the first half of the twentieth century did free women from some of their most challenging tasks, our culture didn't stop to ask questions about these developments. Did *all* these changes really constitute progress? What happens to the way women feel about homemaking when they change from producers of the family's products to consumers? What happens when women must rely on outside experts for advice on everything from what we should eat to how we should treat our children? What happens when we are told to make our routine jobs brainless and we spend the majority of our time in our car? We were to see.

"The Problem That Has No Name": Betty Friedan and *The Feminine Mystique*

In 1963, Betty Friedan fired the opening salvo of the modern women's movement with the publication of her book *The Feminine*

Mystique. In this book, she put into words "the problem that has no name": that women were largely unhappy with the role that our culture prescribed for them. She stated that women needed to be "liberated" from housework in order to fulfill their potential through paid employment. This was a message that resonated with millions of women.

What Friedan articulated was the growing discontent of the American housewife. Interestingly, writer and Nobel Prize laureate Pearl S. Buck made many of the same points about the plight of the American housewife in a book written in 1941. Returning to the United States from China, where she lived for many years, she was astonished to observe that the status of the American woman was so low. Isolated, discouraged from using their minds for anything outside the narrow sphere of the home, and cut off from aspects of homemaking that had taken considerable skill, Buck concluded that American women were "starving at the source." She went on to describe how women had almost no influence on American national life, and how feminine qualities were despised. She also noted, with some alarm, that women were passing this disdain for all things female on to the next generation. She wrote: "What is one to think of women who deliberately teach their sons to despise women?" (Buck 1941, 44)

However, as historian Glenna Matthews suggests, the time was not yet right for women to openly discuss their unhappiness with the changing role of the housewife. America was just recovering from the Great Depression and was soon to enter World War II. Further, the forces that had devalued the work of the housewife didn't reach their full flower until the 1950s.

The 1950s: The Golden Era for Families?

The 1950s have often been described as the "golden era" of the American family. It is true that the majority of women during this time did stay home with their children. But as we have seen, the culture itself did not have positive things to say about women at home. Negative or unattainably perfect stereotypes were reinforced by yet another technological invention: television.

In the meantime, the destruction of mother-to-mother transmission of skills and the constant messages of advertisers had another insidious effect: the loss of skills became real. Women really were forced to rely on goods and services provided by other people, putting us even more firmly in the role of consumers rather than producers—and if we were to believe advertisers, fairly dumb consumers at that. To me, the most troubling aspect of this decline in skills is the financial bondage it places families in. Purchased alternatives are almost always more expensive than what you can do at home. But since we feel we don't have any choice, we continue to purchase expensive goods and services—sometimes teetering at the brink of poverty to do so.

Traditionalists often blame Betty Friedan and other feminists for devaluing homemaking and creating women's unhappiness. This is neither fair nor accurate. Many other forces led to the unhappiness of American housewives. Friedan simply named the problem. However, Matthews, a feminist historian, points out that the early women's movement did make the mistake of adopting our culture's contempt for all things domestic.

Two generations later, women are questioning whether simply shedding all vestiges of the housewife role is really the solution. Many women are working full-time and still doing the bulk of child and home care. Many are asking whether we have traded the bondage of one cultural tradition for another. Can caring for children and tending a home be rewarding activities? Have we, in fact, thrown the baby out with the bath water?

The Rise of Modern Domesticity

Interest in domesticity is once again on the rise. Books on the joys of mothering and making a warm, beautiful home are hitting the bestseller list. Some examples include Sarah Ban Breathnach's *Simple Abundance* (1995), Victoria Moran's *Shelter for the Spirit* (1997), and Alexandra Stoddard's many titles, including *Creating a Beautiful Home* (1992). But the rise of domesticity is perhaps best personified in a single woman.

Martha Stewart: The Return of the Notable Housewife

Business Week magazine dubbed Martha Stewart "America's lifestyle queen," noting that "even those who scoff at Stewart's perfect-housewife image admit that she's a stunningly savvy entrepreneur" (Brady 2000). Her various business enterprises include *Mar-*

tha Stewart Living magazine, a television show, a Web site that racked up record Christmas sales last year, and products for garden and home. She is one of the wealthiest women in America. Clearly, *someone* is buying her products. Diane Fisher (1996) describes why she thinks Stewart's brand of new domesticity is catching on:

> Perhaps many of us, raised in a generation geared up to juggle all the balls—the cellular phone, briefcase, handweights, and diaper bag—perhaps we're finally getting ready to opt out of an inhuman scenario: this idea of doing it all . . . As unreal and perfect as Martha Stewart can be, she reminds us of the joy in arranging flowers, gardening, lovingly setting a table. We are almost ready to admit that we miss the domestic arts! (133)

What I've also found telling, however, is the viciousness of many of the attacks against her, including snide remarks about her ethnic heritage. One spoof called her the "dominatrix of domesticity." Given what we know about history, we should be somewhat troubled by the appearance, once again, of the "housewife bitch." Of course, many people joke about her because she sets the bar so high. But I like the fact that she puts a positive face on domesticity, shows women how to live with style and beauty, and encourages women to learn new skills. Very few mortals could even come close to doing all she does—and we don't have to. My hope is that as we become more confident in our own choices, we can use her as the resource she is, rather than feel inferior because we are not just like her.

Women's Ways of Knowing

There has also been a recent resurgence of interest in "women's ways of knowing." One of the most influential books in this movement is *Toward a New Psychology of Women* (1995) by Jean Baker Miller. The premise of this book, and others that followed it, is that women approach life differently than men. Women's growth and psychological development occurs in relationships with others, including our families and friends. Men tend to be independent; women are more likely to seek relationships. Rather than despising our femaleness, we should embrace it. "Relational" theory resonates with thousands of women.

This willingness to embrace women's history and culture has also led to a resurgence of interest in women's craft traditions, such as quilting, stitchery, and cooking. Indeed, quilts made by traditional groups, such as the Amish, are now recognized as works of art and sell for hundreds of dollars. Older quilts are often worth even more, and are becoming part of museum folk-art collections.

Environmental Concerns

Change may be coming from another source that has little to do with domesticity per se, but could have a large impact on families. With an increasing concern about the environment, many have been calling for a change in the way we consume goods. According to Vicki Robins of the New Road Map Foundation, overconsumption is bad for us in a number of ways. It leads to a declining quality of life. We work longer hours in jobs we may hate so we can buy more stuff. Overconsumption leads to debt, economic weakness, and the lowest savings rate in the world. Finally, overconsumption leads to problems for the environment, including the accumulation of toxic waste and garbage, water and air pollution, and the depletion of renewable resources (Robins 1994).

Waste is a direct result of consumerism. The business practice of "planned obsolescence" generates an enormous amount of waste as manufacturers change colors or styles frequently to get you to continue to buy. This applies to everything from clothing to plastic containers to household appliances (think avocado-green refrigerators).

Noting that massive consumerism is having a negative impact on the environment, two recent summits have convened in Japan on "sustainable consumption," or consumption that does not have a negative environmental impact (Myers 2000). If implemented, policies that resulted from these meetings will have a dramatic impact on our spending habits. These policies could include eliminating subsidies for fossil fuels, foods, and other products, allowing the true (much higher) prices of these items to surface. The new higher prices would curb consumerism and encourage families to abandon the buy-and-dump mentality that is still prevalent in the U.S. If this seems somewhat "leftist" to you, you should know that the staunchly conservative Theodore Roosevelt warned Americans almost 100 years ago that unbridled consumerism would cripple America (Wills 1937).

The Reappearance of the Mother/Activist

As their counterparts in the 1850s did, mothers are once again using the moral authority of their role to call for social changes. There have been many examples in recent years of mother activism. I have selected two. The first example is Mothers Against Drunk Drivers (MADD),which was founded in 1980 by a group of mothers after a thirteen-year-old girl was killed by a drunk driver. At the time MADD was formed, sentences for drunk drivers were lenient. In just a few years this organization managed to change public opinion about the seriousness of drunk driving.

Another example of mother/activism is "The Million Mom March" held in Washington, D.C. on Mother's Day, 2000. In this case, mothers organized around the issue of gun control. To quote from their Web site (www.millionmom.com), their purpose "is to prevent gun death and injury and to support victims of gun trauma. We want common sense gun laws. We want to keep our children and our families safe in a nation that is flooded with unregistered, unlicensed, and unregulated guns." Many of the mothers who participated had husbands or children who were killed with guns.

Like Harriet Beecher Stowe before them, mothers in both of these organizations turn their personal pain into social action, and they do so referring specifically to their role as mothers.

Discourse on Work Options for Mothers

Our discussion has now come full circle. You will recall that we started by acknowledging that women often feel a vague sense of guilt. As you can see, there have been a variety of cultural forces shaping how we live and the choices we make. And not all of these have been benign or had our best interests at heart.

As a mother, you *must* feel free to evaluate your options and make choices based on what's best for your family. In a recent interview, Senator Hillary Rodham Clinton—an icon of the "working mother" since the 1992 presidential election—acknowledged that women should be free to choose whether they stay home with children or seek employment outside the home (Stan 2000):

> I think we should do everything possible to give families real choices about whether or when one or both parents should work during a child's young years, because there isn't any doubt in my mind that the most important job any of us have is caring for children. (63)

I hope that this discussion of our past helps you examine the "shoulds" in your life. It can be enlightening to realize that many of the tasks we do and the standards we have adopted were not freely chosen, but were "given" to us by the advertising industry and an army of experts. To realize the goal of bringing our workload down to a more manageable level, we must begin to make conscious choices about our work at home and in the marketplace—the topic of the next two chapters.

CHAPTER 5

FOR LOVE OR MONEY
WORK ARRANGEMENTS THAT WORK FOR YOU

Mothers at home versus mothers in the workplace: the popular media has been quick to dub the tension between these groups "the mommy wars." To tell the truth, I approach this topic with some hesitation. Everyone, it seems, has an opinion on this subject, and the discussion can indeed get ugly. But employment is a potentially major source of mothering stress. We need to talk about it.

I enter this discussion as someone who has done it all. Since having my kids, I've worked full-time and part-time, I've had a home-based business, and been home full-time. After having all these different roles I've observed two things.

1. No choice is perfect. There are advantages and drawbacks to any arrangement you make.

2. No matter which one you choose, someone will be unhappy with you.

Mothers can be pretty nasty to each other. Neither at-home nor employed mothers can claim moral high ground, either. I've gotten it from both sides, as have many of the other mothers I know.

If your current work arrangement is working for you, you can probably skip ahead to the next chapter. But if you want to explore your options, read on. You might be in search of a schedule with more sanity. You may want to use your skills while being available to your children, or find a way to stay home for a few years. Or you may be a mother at home who is thinking about reentering the workforce. Recognize that while a "perfect solution" is an illusion, a "good solution" is entirely possible.

THE HIDDEN FEELINGS OF MOTHERHOOD

Why Mothers Work

Mothers work for a variety of reasons. Understanding why you work can help you find an arrangement that is best for you.

To Earn Money

Money is the most obvious reason to work, and it is not a trivial issue. If you are single, you work to support your children. The choice is work or public assistance, particularly if child support is sporadic or nonexistent. Even when two members of a family work, you may need both salaries just to make ends meet.

For families with lower incomes, your wages may mean the difference between "making it" and poverty. For example, according to the U.S. Department of Labor (1997b), in families of Hispanic origin, the median income for single mothers was $13,474. For households with only a father, the median is $22,257. For married-couple families, the median family income is $29,861. The statistics are even more striking for black families, where family income varies greatly according to whether the wife is employed. When both husbands and wives were employed, the median family income is $48,533; when the wife was not in the labor force, it is only $25,507. For female-headed households, the median income is $15,004 (U.S. Department if Labor 1997a). Even if your family is not near the poverty level, the second salary gives you a financial buffer that provides security, especially in this era of downsizing. In many parts of the country, a second salary may also be necessary if you want to purchase a house.

From a psychological standpoint, money is important too. Money often equals power in a family. Women may experience a subtle, or not so subtle, shift in the balance of power in their families when they step out of the workforce. Extra home and child care often falls upon the person who makes the least amount of money. Given our culture's lack of respect for at-home mothers, this is hardly surprising.

To Pay Off Debts

An issue related to money is debt. Many mothers work to pay off large debts. Some of these debts were from student loans. Mothers with advanced or professional degrees often feel that they must work to justify the large amount of debt they incurred, or the loans may be their partner's. Credit card and other consumer debt is another source of strain in families. Interest on this type of debt is so expensive that it is often difficult to pay it off. Families can be in bondage to consumer debts for years. Unfortunately, advertisers continue to encourage families to live beyond their means.

To Keep Health Insurance

Another issue related to money is health insurance. Some mothers work because their job has health insurance. To quit their jobs, or even to go part-time, would mean losing their coverage. In families where someone has a preexisting condition, the mother may be afraid to leave an insurer for fear that person won't be covered by a new insurer.

To Experience Satisfaction in a Job Well Done

Mothering is notoriously lacking in indicators of job performance; it may take *years* before you know whether you did a good job as a mother. In contrast, there are often more tangible rewards from paid employment, and the tasks are more concrete, with obvious beginnings and endings. Also, depending on the type of job you have and how long you've been doing it, you may have developed a high level of skill. It's wonderful to have skills and use them. You may not feel very skillful as a mother.

Because You Love Your Work

You may work because you *love* what you do for a living. It may be something that is an integral part of who you are. You work because you couldn't imagine not being able to do the work you love. This was very much an issue for me, and it is for many other mothers I meet.

Because You Crave Intellectual Stimulation

Full-time child care is demanding work, and you may find yourself starved for adult conversation. You may long to continue to learn things, keep up on current events, and pursue culture. Sometimes work can give you these things.

Because Other People Expect You to Work

You may also work because that is what your friends and family expect of you. The pressure to work can be subtle or overt. Some may have told you that you are letting other women down or that you are wasting your education. You may get pressure from your own mother who didn't like being home, or from your husband or partner who wants a higher standard of living.

To Be Different than Your Mother

Growing up, you may have observed your own mother being unhappy at home and were determined not to follow in her footsteps. Even if your mother enjoyed her time at home, you may have unconsciously adopted our culture's contempt for housewives in general, and decided not to do as she did.

To Follow a Career Path

You may also work to keep up with a career. Perhaps you have worked hard to become a member of a profession. You might be a year or two from a specific goal such as finishing a residency, making partner, or getting tenure. You may also have a license that you worked hard to get, and that you want to keep current.

To Escape from Home

You may work because there is chaos at home. You may be overwhelmed by caregiving responsibilities. Maybe your children are difficult to be around. Susan returned to work not only because she was feeling overwhelmed with taking care of her children and aging mother, but also because her house was isolated and dark during much of the day. Being inside all day, especially during the winter, made her feel trapped.

Because You Want to Make a Difference

Finally, mothers work outside the home because they want to make a difference. You may have a cause that you feel strongly about, and don't think you can wait five or ten years to do something about it. Perhaps you have the type of job (such as being a medical doctor or nurse) where the fruits of your labor are dramatic, and you see that you are saving lives. Your job may be less dramatic, but one that still touches people's lives. This is not to say that being home with children doesn't make a difference, for it certainly does. But the results of your efforts at home are long-term and may not have the immediate results that working in your field does.

How Much Does It Cost You to Work?

The next thing to consider is how much it costs you to work. Sometimes we only take into account the most obvious expenses, such as day care, but there are many others you may not have thought of. On the surface, it may seem you are getting ahead. But as you calculate your true cost of working, you might actually find that you are losing money when you work.

The figure you need to know is how much you have left after you have covered all your work-related expenses—how much you are "netting." When you know this figure, you may become open to more options. As we just discussed, there are lots of reasons for working, and money is only one of them. But if you realize you are actually *losing* money, perhaps you can come up with an arrangement that is less costly in terms of both money and your physical and mental energy.

If there are two of you working, consider how much it costs each of you to work. You and your partner might decide that it makes more sense for you to stay in your job while your partner stays home with the kids. If you want some help in calculating how much the second income brings in, check out the "second income calculator" at msn.com.

Increase in Tax Rate

You might be surprised to learn that this can be your biggest expense. Your salary might be just enough to push you into a higher tax bracket. I was stunned to learn that 48 percent of my full-time salary went to taxes. From the money that was left, we still had to pay all the other expenses, like day care for two kids. However, I discovered that my salary from part-time work did not raise our tax rate. By working part-time, I was netting almost the same that I would have for full-time work, but with a greatly reduced level of stress.

Child Care

Child care is the next-largest expense. Child care can be cost-effective when you have one child. But child-care costs for two or more children can be prohibitively expensive. Finding quality day care that you can afford continues to be one of the toughest challenges mothers who are employed face.

Commuting

In chapter 1, I described the costs of commuting in terms of time and stress. Now let's talk money. The IRS allows $.345 a mile as the cost of business travel. Use this figure to calculate how much your commute costs, realizing that it is probably on the low side. Be sure to include any tolls and parking fees that you pay. Also recognize that commuting costs are going to keep going up as fuel costs continue to rise. If you use public transit, calculate the amount you pay on a weekly or monthly basis.

Clothing

No question about it, when you are employed outside the home, you will probably need nicer clothes than when you are at home. Different occupations have different standards. Someone working in a law office will have to dress up more than someone in a manufacturing job. Be sure to include any hosiery, makeup, salon, or accessory expenses here too.

Purchase of Services

When mothers are employed, families purchase more services. The obvious one is day care. You may also purchase more meals out and more convenience and take-out foods. You might hire out house cleaning, gardening, car washing, and dog walking. There is nothing wrong with hiring help you need. In fact, I suggest it in the next chapter. But when calculating the costs of employment outside the home, these costs must be included.

Purchase of "Treats"

When you feel stressed, it is often easy to justify the purchase of treats for yourself or your children because you are working so hard.

These treats can range from large to small, from snack foods to jewelry to a really nice car. Again, how you spend your money is your business. But you should realize that you are more likely to make expensive purchases when you are employed.

Creating Work That's Right for You

In this section, I describe some basic work options. The type of work you actually do will vary, but there are many options that you may have never considered. Sometimes mothers are hesitant to ask for "special" privileges just on the basis of their child-care needs. It's important to stand back and look at the big picture. More and more people are calling for work options, and not just for reasons of parenting. People are asking for reduced hours to improve the quality of their lives through volunteering or other meaningful activity. People are asking for flexible work options so that they can care for aging parents or be with a child who is having difficulties. People with disabilities find that work options allow them to participate in the workforce rather than relying totally on public assistance. More-

---

ARE MEN THE BEST ROLE MODELS?

We tend to think that work and family dilemmas are only for women. Men, we feel, never have to make these kinds of choices and sacrifices. But is that really true? Would our lives be better if we had a "wife" at home to take care of things?

In his book *The Paradox of Success* (1993), former businessman John O'Neil describes his climb up the corporate ladder. He was always traveling, making big deals, being really important. One morning, as he was leaving for a trip, his young daughter was clinging to his legs, begging him not to go. The limo driver who had come to pick him up didn't say a word, but gave him a look of disapproval in the rearview mirror. Even years later, that look still got under his skin. He cites that incident as when he first started to question whether he really had his priorities straight. I found the subtitle of his book telling: *When Winning at Work Means Losing at Life*. Before we uncritically adopt a male model of success, we should at least consider what men who have done it that way have to say about their lives.

---

over, working from home, flexible schedules, and compressed work weeks lead to less traffic in congested areas and are generally better for the environment.

Telecommuting and Web-based businesses are opening up opportunities for people in small or geographically isolated communities, many of which have costs of living that are substantially less than living in a city. Virtual work boosts local economies in small towns and rural areas as telecommuters and people with Web-based businesses move to these areas. Our little state of New Hampshire (population 1.1 million) has the highest per capita rate of workers in high-tech in the country. Work alternatives are catching on.

The Demographic Imperative

In *Breaking with Tradition: Women and Work, the New Facts of Life* (1992), Felice Schwartz describes the "demographic imperative" that will force companies to make some changes. The future workforce will have fewer white males than ever before, so companies that want to hire and retain competent staffs will have to look to women, minorities, and (I would add) people with disabilities. Schwartz sees greater opportunities for these disenfranchised parts of the workforce than ever before. And if companies want to include women of child-bearing age, they'll need to recognize some practical adaptations.

Below, I've listed some of the major types of work options. These can be combined any number of different ways in a two-adult household. My husband and I both telecommute, and have for many years. I've also had a variety of nontraditional work arrangements.

Flex-Time and Compressed Work Weeks

"Flex-time" refers to starting and finishing work at nonstandard times. It might mean starting early and leaving early, or starting late and working later in the day. For some types of jobs, this type of scheduling is not possible. But when it is, it might let you meet the school bus, get to work before commuter traffic is in full swing, or accommodate a longer morning routine.

A similar concept is the compressed work week, wherein a full work week is compressed into four ten-hour days, or three twelve-hour days. This allows for more full days at home, but with full-time benefits.

Part-time

Part-time work is another popular option. The number of hours can vary tremendously, from a few hours a week to almost full-time. Sometimes, employees share their jobs with another person, or function as independent contractors who are employed hourly or on a contract basis. Part-time positions are generally not advertised, but many types of work can be adapted to fit a part-time schedule. Part-time work is also attractive to employers since it is often cheaper to hire a part-time worker or independent contractor than a full-time employee. Organizations like the Association of Part-time Professionals can give you suggestions on how to arrange for part-time work.

Telecommuting

Telecommuting is an increasingly popular alternative work arrangement. It can be full- or part-time, and involves working at home while communicating with your employer via telephone, fax, and e-mail. You can telecommute for all or part of your work week. My husband, Doug, has telecommuted full-time for over twelve years. He works for a high-tech company in southern California. We live in New Hampshire, in a town of 3,200. Both of us started telecommuting before it was trendy, and people told us that it would never work. It does.

Home- or Web-based Business

Another alternative is to start your own business. According to the Business Women's Network, by 2005 there will be an estimated 4.7 million self-employed women in the workforce. That's an increase of 77 percent. You can start almost any type of business: you can make things to sell, publish information, or be involved with a reputable multilevel marketing business. The woman who cuts my hair also sells antiques over the Internet. A local coffee company has a small retail outlet, but also sells its unique "New Hampshire" blends all over the world (check them out at www.nhcoffeeroasters.com).

If you have professional skills, you can also sell your time as a consultant and provide training to people in your field. If you have office or computer skills, you may hire yourself out as a "virtual" assistant. There is increasing demand for people who will help other entrepreneurs from remote locations, usually via the Internet. For lots of ideas on home-based businesses, check out *Homemade Money* (1997) by Barbara Brabec.

> The old joke that a person's job was replaced by a computer has given way to a new truism: A person and her computer are replacing the corporation.
>
> (from *Working Mother* magazine)

Sequencing

Sequencing is another option for making a manageable lifestyle. Its name is taken from a book entitled (oddly enough) *Sequencing* (1996) by Arlene Cardozo. Sequencing takes that long view of your life and says you can "have it all, but not all at the same time." The idea is that you have a time when you concentrate on your career. Then you step out of the workforce for a few years to raise your children.

When your children are in school, or are a little more independent, you return to the workforce. Of all the books I've read, this one offers the most specific suggestions for keeping up your career while tending your children. For example, Cardozo advises mothers to keep up their professional licenses, stay involved in their professional organizations, and stay up on their fields. While you have young children at home, she suggests that you limit your work week to ten hours, and that you don't take assignments with tight deadlines. That way, you still have the flexibility that you need to respond to your children's needs.

Sequencing can also be a helpful approach if you need to take an extended leave due to a health or other crisis in your family. On two separate occasions, I have had to take a six-month leave due to lupus flares. On both of these occasions, I could not work at all. Using the sequencing model, I kept up with my reading. The added psychological benefit was that sequencing kept me from becoming depressed and gave me a vision of life beyond being sick.

Advantages of Alternative Work Arrangements

Besides giving you more control over your schedule, alternative work arrangements offer some advantages that you might not have considered.

Tax Advantages

Both telecommuting and home-based businesses offer lots of nice tax advantages. Your home office must be your primary workspace. But if it is, you can take a percentage of all home expenses you incur over the year off your taxes. For example, if your home office is about 20 percent of your home, you can deduct 20 percent of your electric bill, gas bill, and other home maintenance costs from your taxes. While your apparent take-home pay may be substantially less when you work for yourself, you should be sure to include these hefty tax savings when comparing how much you are netting at home versus outside work.

Caution, however, is in order. If you are self-employed, you will have to pay "self-employment" tax—the portion of Social Security your employer would normally cover. This can be a substantial cost. Be sure to check with your accountant or tax preparer to find out the most current tax laws regarding home offices before taking any deductions. Home-office deductions can flag you for an audit, so keep *all* receipts related to home care.

Reduced Costs of Working

Alternative work arrangements allow you to substantially cut your cost of working. Your commuting costs will often be less and, if you work at home, your clothing cost will usually be substantially less. You can also reduce the cost of lunches out.

One cost that you will probably reduce, but not entirely eliminate, is child care. If you are working at home, you will probably still need some. Even a few hours every week can give you a chance to concentrate on paperwork or return phone calls. And you can often have your provider right in your home so you are available if need be.

More Flexibility

Alternative working arrangements also give you a chance to be more involved in your children's lives. If the school nurse calls, you can go retrieve your child from school. You can take an afternoon off to see a school play or help in a classroom. You can run errands or schedule appointments during the day so that these are not all left for the weekend. These work arrangements offer you a lot more control over your life.

Modeling for Your Children

If you work at home, your children can actually see what you do for a living. It gets them more involved in your life and shows them "work in action." It also shows them someone who is successfully balancing work and family. As they get older, you might even hire them to do some work for you.

Alternative Work Arrangements Are Good for Business

Companies that allow for flexible work options also benefit. Employees are happier on the job and are therefore less susceptible to stress-related illness. This lowers healthcare costs. Employees with alternative arrangements are more productive. Companies are better able to retain employees, reducing costly turnover. When the job market is tight, companies that are truly family-friendly will have an advantage in attracting new talent.

Some Drawbacks of Alternative Work Arrangements

As I mentioned before, there are drawbacks to almost any arrangement you can make. There is no perfect arrangement, but by anticipating some of the possible problems, you can often head them off.

Invisibility

When you are not in your office every day, or at normal times, you can become invisible to your coworkers. You may get passed over for assignments, miss meeting announcements, and generally feel out of the loop. This can be a problem, especially if you are on a specific career path.

There are several approaches you can take. First, be sure that your boss is aware of what you are doing with regular contacts and progress reports. Keeping the lines of communication open with coworkers really helps. Perhaps a colleague feels that he or she must pick up the slack for you. There may be something you can do to remedy this situation. Having a contact in your office can keep you abreast of what's going on and remind others of your existence. Try to cultivate such allies, and let them know that you appreciate them on a regular basis.

You might also need to go to your office periodically. David, a local computer programmer, works at home four days a week and spends a fifth day in his main office. My husband goes into his office in California about four times a year. Note: If you do have two regular offices, it can affect your home-office status with regard to tax deductions.

Perception of Others

In some corporate cultures, someone who wants to work less than sixty (or seventy or eighty) hours a week is suspect. In *The Time Bind* (1997), Arlie Hochschild's respondents indicated that even in a company with family-friendly policies in place, there was often subtle, or even overt, pressure not to take advantage of these policies.

In my own life, I was surprised to learn that even serious illness was not an adequate reason, in some people's minds, for not working "enough." Realizing that some people are really unreasonable about how much they think everyone else should work was surprisingly freeing. I also figured out that my work arrangements are no one else's business.

With a compressed work week or flextime arrangement, you may find that people don't approve when you leave earlier than they do, or don't come in one or two days a week. Your boss may call meetings after your normal quitting time. You may feel pressured to stay, even though you started your day hours before everyone else.

If you have an alternative work arrangement, you may find yourself taken off of projects or "mommy-tracked." Julie, a junior faculty member at a major university, was told that her department expected long hours from her if she was to get tenure. Her work was excellent, but she wanted to be home with her family in the evening. Her solution? She slipped over to her office each evening, turned on the light, locked her office door—and went home! She was recently awarded tenure.

You may not want to resort to that kind of subterfuge. And only you can determine how seriously you want to take other people's attempts to track you. Keep in mind that eventually people get used to these arrangements. If you keep turning in excellent work, people in your office will get the message that you are working hard too. But if you find that you are getting seriously undermined, remember why you wanted an alternative work arrangement in the first place, and then make some positive changes. If it is a big deal, challenge it.

If you can't fix it, ignore it or consider leaving. Being constantly undermined will eventually affect your well-being.

Finally, some people will be jealous of your work arrangements and will let you know it. It's best to respond in a nondefensive but honest way to these verbal missiles. When people say "It must be nice," say "It is." When they say "You're lucky," say "Luck had very little to do with it." When people say "I wish I had that kind of job," say "I'm confident that you could." These kinds of answers deflect sarcastic remarks without justifying your arrangements to others. Remember, you don't owe every nosy person an explanation about your work. If someone sincerely wants to know, I'll share information. Otherwise, I consider particulars about my working arrangements to be private.

Isolation

Just as isolation is a problem for the at-home mother, it also can be for someone working at home. It's important that you get out of the house occasionally, even if it is to take a walk or run some errands. Make sure that you are not sitting in front of your computer every day with no outside human contact. When you start losing your social skills or spending all day in your pajamas, it may be time to get more involved in the outside world.

You must also realistically consider your temperament. Are you someone who likes to work alone? Do you mind being by yourself for long stretches of time? If you like to have other people around, working at home full-time may not be for you.

Lack of Demarcation between Home and Work

Another real danger is that you may actually end up working *more* with an alternative work situation. Part-timers know that hours can multiply until they are working close to full-time (often for part-time pay). Having your work at home, especially, makes it difficult to draw a line between the two. It's very easy to slip into a home office at all hours of the day or night. You may work through mealtimes and into the wee hours of the morning. My husband's company is in California (meaning a three-hour time difference), and it's not unusual for us to receive phone calls at eight or even nine o'clock at night. If at all possible, have a separate work telephone line and office. When it's time to quit for the day, close the door and turn off the phone ringer. Sometimes that's hard to do, but you must draw this line if you want your arrangement to continue to work for you.

Another work/family line is teaching family members to respect your working time. While you want to be available, you also need to let people know that there are times when you need to concentrate on work. Having a separate space to work that is off limits to others can be a challenge if you live in a small apartment or house. Space is one more factor in considering alternative working arrangements.

What You Can Do

Since I have an unusual working situation, I'm often asked how I arranged it. Both my husband and I have learned some things through trial and error. Here are some suggestions I give to mothers who are looking for work alternatives.

Imagine Your Ideal Job

Approach the question of employment with an open mind. Over the years, I've been amazed at the creative choices that families have made, including different shifts, fathers home full-time, and both partners working part-time. I've heard of mothers who are mail carriers, whose day care facility is on their route. This allows them to see their children at lunch.

If you approach every possibility with a "yes, but. . . ," you dramatically limit your ability to come up with a solution. Take a moment and think about what your ideal life would look like, and don't stop yourself with "yes, buts . . ." In your ideal life, what type of work and how much of it would you do? How would you get to and from work? What type of child-care arrangements would you make (including staying home yourself)? Consider writing these ideas down. Often, this exercise can help us pinpoint areas of our lives that contribute to our stress levels.

Be sure to go back to the list earlier in this chapter about why we work. Which of these reasons are important to you? Are there ways that you can incorporate them into a new working arrangement?

Realistically Assess How Much You Are Netting Now

Figure out how much you are actually netting in your current job. Even if money is your primary reason for working, you might find that you can gross a lot less than you are now, and still be netting the same. Also, consider whether you can live on less. Two great books to help you do that are Amy Dacyczyn's *The Tightwad Gazette* (all three volumes) and Dominguez and Robin's *Your Money or Your Life* (1992). These books will give you lots of suggestions about really saving money and improving the quality of your life at the same time.

Consider Leaving Your Current Company

You may find that your current employer is unwilling to make accommodations for you. If that is true, you might consider seeking another job. Again, research your options. If you don't know where to begin, take a look at *Working Mother* magazine. Each year they publish a listing of family-friendly companies—complete with contact information. Also, the library is a great source for books on all types of working arrangements. Sometimes, just knowing that you *could* leave may make your current situation more bearable.

Develop a Plan

If you want a livable working arrangement, assume that you will have to take the initiative. While companies may eventually catch on and offer these options on their own, it may take years. Research your options and present a plan. Try to anticipate the concerns of current or prospective employers, and tell them how you will address those concerns. For example, my husband's current employer was concerned about hiring someone who lived so far away. He offered to work for them on a trial basis for three months. That was seven years ago.

Don't Rush into Change

In some cases, the change you make may be dramatic. Your plan has a much higher probability of success if it's not one that was made on impulse. Cautionary tales abound of men and women leaving their high-powered jobs to open a little store or country inn—only to be miserable in their new lives. Even with a plan, you might still find yourself in culture shock. But chances are you'll be happier with your new arrangement if you've had some time to think it through and weigh your many possible options.

Be Confident

Confidence is contagious. Project it to prospective or current employers, even if you have to fake it at first. You don't have to apologize for wanting "special arrangements." Many other people want them too. You could be a role model for other women. Be confident that you have unique skills to offer. Be honest about your needs and limitations, and present a positive plan for how you will deal with them. Realize too that not everyone will be willing to make these types of accommodations. If they don't, talk to someone else. Remember, alternative work arrangements are good for employers too.

For Further Reading

Resources for Alternative Work Arrangements

These books are full of ideas on different work arrangements. Read them with an open mind. You might be amazed at what you come up with.

Arden, L., J. T. Moyle, and B. Hurwitz. 1999. *The Work-at-Home Sourcebook.* Palo Alto, Calif.: Live Oak Publications.

Brabec, B. 1997. *Homemade Money: How to Select, Start, Manage, Market and Multiply the Profits of a Business at Home.* Cincinnati: F & W Publications.

Bredim, A., and K. K. Lagatree. 1998. *The Home-office Solution: How to Balance your Professional and Personal Lives While Working at Home.* New York: John Wiley & Sons.

Cardozo, A. R. 1996. *Sequencing: A New Solution for Women Who Want Marriage, Career and Family.* San Bernardino, Calif.: Borgo Press.

Folger, L. 2000. *The Stay-at-Home Mom's Guide to Making Money.* Roseville, Calif.: Prima Communications.

Igbaria, M., and M. Tan. 1998. *The Virtual Workplace.* Hershey, Penn.: Idea Group Publishing.

Levin, M. R. 1998. *Teleworking and Urban Development Patterns: Goodbye Uglyville—Hello Paradise.* Lanham, Md.: University Press of America.

Nilles, J. M. 1998. *Managing Telework: Strategies for Managing the Virtual Workforce.* New York: John Wiley & Sons.

Parlapiano, E. H., and C. P. Cobe. 1996. *Mompreneur: A Mother's Step-by-Step Guide to Work-at-Home Success.* New York: Berkley Publishing.

Roberts, L. M. 1997. *How to Raise a Family and a Career Under One Roof.* Moon Township, Penn.: Bookhaven Press.
Association of Part-time Professionals: 703-684-6963
Families and Work Institute: www.familiesandwork.org
Independent Home Workers Alliance: www.homeworkers.org
Information on options Ridewise/Workwise: find at www.ridewise. org/programs/workwise.htm
9 to 5, National Association for Working Women: 800-522-0925
Mother's Home Business Network: www.homeworkingmom.com
Babycenter.com: find referrals and links to other organizations at www.babycenter.com/workandfamily/
Telecommuting Knowledge Center: www.telecommuting.org

Books Describing the Work/Family Dilemma

These two books do a good job of summarizing the issues and dilemmas for employed and at-home mothers. They both offer information on alternative work arrangements and present lots of mothers' stories.

Lewis, D. S., and C. C. Yoest. 1996. *Mother in the Middle: Searching for Peace in the Mommy Wars.* New York: HarperCollins.
Marshall, M. M. 1991. *Good Enough Mothers.* Princeton, N.J.: Peterson's.

Resources for Money and Debt

If you are thinking you'd like to stay home or explore working fewer hours, these books will give very specific suggestions on how to live on less—usually with greatly increased satisfaction. *Your Money or Your Life* has a great guide to calculating what your real hourly wage is.

Dacyczyn, A. 1992. *The Tightwad Gazette.* New York: Villard Books.
———. 1995. *The Tightwad Gazette II.* New York: Villard Books.
———. 1996. *The Tightwad Gazette III.* New York: Villard Books.
Dominguez, J., and V. Robin. 1992. *Your Money or Your Life: Transforming Your Relationship with Money and Achieving Financial Independence.* New York: Viking.
Strauss, S. D., and P. Sander. 2000. *The Complete Idiot's Guide to Beating Debt.* New York: MacMillan
Simple Living Network: www.slnet.com
New Road Map Foundation: www.slnet.com/cip/nrm
National Foundation for Credit Counseling: www.nfcc.org
National Center for Financial Education: www.ncfe.org

Resources for Employed Mothers

These books offer support and advice to mothers who are employed. Guilt for employed mothers is described, as are strategies to counteract it. Alternative work arrangements are also described here as well.

Galinsky, E. 1999. *Ask the Children: What America's Children Really Think about Working Parents.* New York: William Morrow & Company.
Garey, A. L. 1999. *Weaving Work and Motherhood.* Philadelphia: Temple University Press.
Goldman, K. W. 1998. *Working Mothers 101: How to Organize Your Life, Your Children, and Your Career to Stop Feeling Guilty and Start Enjoying It All.* New York: HarperTrade.
Marshall, M. M. 1991. *Good Enough Mothers.* Princeton, N.J.: Peterson's.
Pryor, G. 1997. *Nursing Mother, Working Mother.* Boston: The Harvard Common Press.
Weisberg, A. C., and C. A. Buckler. 1994. *Everything a Working Mother Needs to Know.* New York: Doubleday.
Families and Work Institute: www.familiesandwork.org
9 to 5, National Association for Working Women: 800-522-0925
Working Mother magazine: www.workingmother.com

Resources for At-Home Mothers

Unfortunately, many women who are home full-time feel the sting of disapproval. Here are some books, publications, and organizations that can help women at home feel confident in their choice.

Hunter, B. 1991. *Home by Choice: Understanding the Enduring Effects of a Mother's Love.* Sisters, Ore.: Multnomah Books.
Fox, I., and N. M. Lobsenz. 1996. *Being There: The Benefits of a Stay-at-Home Parent.* Hauppauge, N.Y.: Barron's Educational Services.
Friberg, S. 1979. *Every Child's Birthright: In Defense of Mothering.* New York: Bantam Books. This wonderful book is out of print, but many libraries have it.
Jones, F., and A. Jones. 1998. *Come Home to Your Family: How Families Can Survive and Thrive on One Income.* Buffalo, N.Y.: General Distribution Services, Inc.
Ramming, C. 1996. *A Mother's Work: A Guilt-Free Guide for the Stay-at-Home Mom.* New York: Avon Books.
La Leche League International: www.lalecheleague.org
Mothering magazine: www.mothering.com
National Association of At-Home Mothers: www.athomemothers.com

CHAPTER 6

LESS WORK FOR MOTHER
LIGHTENING YOUR LOAD AT HOME

Forty years ago, Betty Friedan wrote that women need to be liberated from housework. Looking at our lives now, I have to ask: Have women been liberated from housework? I think you know the answer. The type of work mothers do has dramatically changed over the past 100 years. However, the sheer number of hours that women devote to child and home care has remained constant, ranging from forty-nine to fifty-six hours a week (Schor 1992). What's going on? Why are mothers continuing to work so hard?

In some ways, it's easy to see why mothers work hard at home. Home is where you feed and clothe your family, nurture your relationships, exercise and sleep, and entertain yourself. Home is where you handle the mountain of paperwork that comes through your hands each day. It is where you launch projects, celebrate special occasions, and offer hospitality to guests. Mothers are shouldering most of this load.

In this chapter, I describe some of the factors that contribute to women's work at home. I encourage you to examine your household routines; making improvements in this area can dramatically improve your life.

Mothers and the Second Shift

When I was in college, we learned that men and women should share child and home care. Nobody thought this was a bad idea; in fact, my classmates, would probably still say the same thing. The reality in many homes, however, is much different. Men do far less at home than women, even when the wives are employed outside the home. Sometimes couples start out equally sharing the work, only to fall into rigid sex roles after having children.

In *The Second Shift* (1989), Arlie Hochshild found that employed women were still doing the majority of the housework and child care. The "second shift" refers to the work they do once they are home (the "first shift" is their jobs). Mothers who are employed often come home to dirty houses, piles of laundry, and hungry families.

A more recent study demonstrated that home is a haven for men, but not for women with children. Researchers compared blood pressures for employed men with children and employed women with children. Men's blood pressure was higher at work than at home. However, women's blood pressure was the same at home as it was at work. (Marco et al. 2000)

At-home mothers also face a second shift. Mothers with young children spend much of their day tending to the needs of the kids; those with children participating in extracurricular activities may find that much of their day is spent in the car. Some days, it's an accomplishment just to take a shower and get dressed. When her partner comes home, an at-home mom often uses this time to prepare dinner, do the laundry, go grocery shopping, or clean the house.

Single mothers have an even larger second shift. They face the huge workload of raising children, being the breadwinner, and caring for a home alone. Single mothers, in particular, can feel overwhelmed by all the tasks that need to be done.

The Paradox of the Laborsaving Device

In Chapter 4, I described what the advent of laborsaving devices did to women's work at home. These machines were supposed to free up lots of time for mothers. What we now realize, of course, is that these devices simply changed the nature of the work without necessarily reducing the time it takes to accomplish the task. Ruth Schwartz Cowan, in *More Work for Mother* (1983), gives perhaps the best analysis of why machines do not necessarily free up time. I will share three of her examples.

The first example is the stove. When women cooked on an open hearth, meals were relatively simple. Women did the cooking, but men and children split and gathered the firewood. When wood cookstoves became the norm, women still cooked but men only needed to provide half the wood. "Stoves were laborsaving devices, but the labor they saved was male" (61). Once gas and electric stoves were introduced, men's participation in cooking completely disappeared, but women still cooked. Moreover, since it was now possible to cook several things at once, meals became more complex and women spent more time overall cooking.

The second example concerns clothing. The advent of mass-produced cloth meant that women no longer needed to spin. Men no longer needed to weave nor children to card. But women still needed to sew. Middle-class women hired seamstresses or had servants who assisted in sewing, but with the advent of the sewing machine, these women began sewing for their families alone. Once manufactured clothing was widely available, women were the ones primarily responsible for the purchase and upkeep of their families' clothing. Now, time is spent shopping, taking items to the dry cleaners, washing, mending, and ironing.

The refrigerator also had an impact on women's daily work. Women no longer needed to shop every day and men no longer needed to haul ice. But the refrigerator put door-to-door vendors out of business. Women began going to large self-service supermarkets, spending more time to shop and to travel to and from the store. When the new Wal-Mart Superstore opened near us, everyone complained because it was now "four miles" to the cash register. A "quick" shopping trip is no longer possible in such a large store.

Finally, Schwartz Cowan points out that although some of women's tasks have changed, women are still responsible for cooking meals, tending children, nursing the sick, and buying and maintaining clothing—a fact little changed by the forces of industrialization. Laborsaving devices do not necessarily save time, but they increase our expectations of what mothers should accomplish.

Chances are, you put in many hours on home and child care. The rest of this chapter, offers some suggestions to help bring your workload to a more manageable level. I recommend three strategies: analyze what you are doing and eliminate any unnecessary tasks; streamline tasks that remain; and share the load with other people, including your partner, your children, and professionals.

Analyze and Eliminate Tasks

Let's start at the beginning, by examining how you spend your time at home. Are there any tasks that you can eliminate? Before you say "no," keep an open mind. Creative solutions often come after a period of brainstorming, when you uncritically consider all possible ideas.

Inventory Your Activities

Start by paying attention to all the activities that fill your days. Focus particularly on activities that take a lot of time. You might want to write a list or keep a log. If you're not sure where to start, take a look at the list in chapter 3 (under "Impossible Job"). Mothers always have a huge "to do" list, and what they accomplish is dwarfed by what they still need to do. But when you write it down, I suspect you will be amazed at how much you actually do accomplish.

Once you have your list in hand, consider each activity and ask yourself whether it needs to be done. If you say "yes" to every item, try another approach. Ask yourself what would be the worst thing that could happen if you didn't do it. The answers may surprise you.

You should also include "kid things" on this list. Mothers want to let their children participate in activities that will make them well-rounded and give them future opportunities. But in many communities, extracurricular activities have gotten way out of hand. Mothers can spend every night of the week driving to lessons, sport practices and games, and other activities. The amount of time involved grows as you add children.

You might seriously consider limiting the number of outside activities your children participate in. It will save you time, and also help your children learn to strike a balance between "enough" and "too much." Relationships in your family can improve when you actually have time to talk with each other instead of rushing off each afternoon or evening.

The choices you make are personal. The solution that works well for my family may not work for yours. I've even found that what worked for me five years ago no longer works because the needs of my family have changed. Realize too that deciding to eliminate an obligation from your list doesn't necessarily mean that you have to eliminate it *today*. For example, your children may be participating in several activities. They may need to finish out the season before they withdraw. I encourage you to be flexible and experiment to find solutions you can live with.

Develop Realistic Standards: Aim for "Clean Enough"

Another area where you can probably eliminate some tasks is in housecleaning. Like anything else, cleanliness can be taken too far. Your home is for you and your family to *live* in. I recommend that you make your home "clean enough." What does that mean? After a certain point, cleanliness is largely a matter of preference. I suggest you use two criteria to hit a level that is good for you. The first criterion is level of organization. Can you find what you need without thrashing around? Do bills get paid on time? Is there an orderly flow of mail and other paper? Do you have a way to track appointments for your family? Can you consistently find your keys, clean underwear, or your glasses? Are you usually well-stocked on items like toilet paper, toothpaste, or milk?

The second criterion is level of cleanliness. A certain minimum standard is necessary for health and safety. After that, "clean" is also subjective. If you invite people over, are you able to relax and enjoy them, or do you wish they would turn around so you can vacuum the rug? Does it take days to get your home in shape for guests? If so, you are unlikely to have company (and you'll be too exhausted to enjoy them). Don Aslett's book *No Time to Clean* (2000) has a section on cleaning tasks you can eliminate, if you need additional suggestions.

If you are cleaning and organizing beyond the point of "clean enough," you can probably do less. On the other hand, if you answered "no" to a lot of these questions, you might be playing catch-up much of the time, or losing time searching for missing items. If that is true for you, the next step will help.

Streamline Your Tasks

Once you have eliminated some tasks, consider whether the ones that are left could be done more efficiently. In most cases, the answer is probably "yes." The good news is that organizational skills can be learned. I spent many years of my adult life being "domestically challenged." It wasn't until my second son was born that I realized I needed to learn some basic household organization strategies. If I can learn, so can you. Below are some steps to get you started. I would also encourage you to read some of the books listed at the end of this chapter for more detailed suggestions.

Analyze the Situation

According to professional organizer Julie Morgenstern (1998), the first step in any organizational scheme is to figure out where you're having problems. Are you always losing keys? Is your morning routine a disaster? Do you buy duplicates when you can't find stuff or because you don't realize what you have? For me, a recent problem was how to handle the flow of mail. Pick your worst situation, and start there first. Don't be tempted to say "everything."

Once you've figured out what you want to change, try mentally walking through the problem to see if you can come up with a solution. If you lose your keys, think about what door you usually use when you come into your home. Would it help if you had a key rack right next to that door? If you tend to have lots of books and magazines next to your bed, would a bookshelf or end table with drawers help? Think about what you *actually* do now rather than what you "should" do. If your organizational efforts are based on shoulds, you'll find that you do not use the system you devised.

Get Rid of Clutter

Clutter can dramatically increase the time you spend cleaning. It takes longer to clean if every surface is covered with knickknacks, and your rooms are overflowing with furniture. Other tasks take longer too. Working in a crammed kitchen is unpleasant and wastes time. Trying to put clothes away in a too-full dresser drawer is a pain. Adding more toys to the three-foot mound is frustrating.

Look around. Is it time to get rid of some possessions? I'm not suggesting you give away your favorite things or your memories. But are there items that are broken? Can they be fixed, or do they need to be replaced or even eliminated? Are there items you don't need that someone else can use? Do you have clothing in four different sizes in your closet?

As you get rid of clutter, I want to alert you to a pitfall that can undermine your efforts. Julie Morgenstern calls it "zigzagging." You start going through a drawer, only to find a book that belongs on the bookshelf. You discover the bookshelf is a mess. You start working on it, discover something that belongs upstairs. So you return that to where it belongs. Next thing you know, you're working on the closet in your bedroom. By day's end, you have half-completed projects all over the house, but haven't finished anything! Instead, try tackling one project at a time. When you find stuff that belongs elsewhere, set it aside in a box. When you have *finished* the project you were working on, take the accumulated items and put them away. In the process, note any other areas that need your attention. One of these might be your next organization project. There are many excellent books to help you declutter, but my all-time favorite is Don Aslett's *Clutter's Last Stand* (1984).

Respect Your Work Spaces

Respecting your work spaces will make it faster and easier for you to work, and will encourage others to work too. Pay particular attention to the kitchen and laundry area, but the principles apply to any area of your home. Basically, by thinking through the kind of work that takes place there, you can make any work spaces more suited to your needs.

First, eliminate all clutter in your work areas. The kitchen is often a place that gets really "decorated." Resist this temptation. Try to keep your counters clear, and be judicious about wall decorations. The kitchen and bath have lots of moist heat that combines with dust to make guck. Everything in these rooms should be very cleanable.

The laundry area often becomes the depository of loose change, missing socks, odds and ends of clothing, and pocket contents. Have a trash can handy, and a bin for transporting loose articles to other places in the house. Also, try to arrange this space so you have somewhere to fold clothes; if you can, it will make laundry much easier for you.

Second, make sure everything you need is at hand. Any job becomes more onerous when it is accompanied by frantic searching. It's also easier to procrastinate, or never do something, if you have to go to another room to get what you need. Think about the supplies and tools you need in each area, and make sure that they are available.

Third, think about your physical comfort. Is there enough light? We think about lighting a lot more in kitchens, but laundry areas frequently have very poor light. Adequate light will make your work area more pleasant and your work easier to do. Consider temperature. Is the area too hot or too cold? Your work will seem much more pleasant if you are a comfortable temperature. Also, if you are doing lots of standing, especially on a cement slab or tiled floor, think about getting an antifatigue mat from a janitor supply store. This can make a very big difference in how your legs and back feel.

Make It Easy to Clean

Since cleaning can occupy a significant portion of your time, you owe it to yourself to make it as easy as possible. One strategy is to keep your cleaning supplies where you need them. If, when it's time to clean the bathroom, for example, you have to make a special trip to the "cleaning closet," guess what happens? You put it off. But if you have your supplies handy, you can take a quick pass and be finished in a few minutes. You'll find that you can use little odd bits of time, like during commercials, rather than needing to dedicate special time to "cleaning the bathroom." Similarly, keep vacuums near where you need them. If you live in a multistory house, you might consider a vacuum for each floor. I also keep cleaning supplies I use for my car in my car. I can use little bits of time to keep the inside of my car clean, and rarely have to set aside special time for this purpose.

Using good-quality cleaning supplies makes an amazing difference. For very little money, you can get supplies that will save you hours, including concentrated cleaners you mix yourself, window squeegees, a good vacuum, and decent cleaning rags. This is another way to respect your work space. Your time is too valuable to waste it using substandard tools, especially those you use every day. Fortunately, well-made cleaning tools are relatively inexpensive in janitor supply stores or over the Internet and will pay you back manyfold.

Finally, consider whether you really need to clean as much as you do. Truth be told, most of the time cleaning too much is not our problem. But there might be areas where you do too much. Sometimes, the best solution is to not clean at all, or to do it less frequently. You might think about replacing things in your house that seem to need a lot of care.

Is Housework Beneath You?

A century's worth of denigrating domestic work has had an insidious effect. Many young women I meet are of the opinion that housework is beneath them. They assume that housework is not for "smart" women, and one way to show that you are smart is to be domestically challenged. These young women rightly reject the image of the woman at home who obsesses about whether her sheets are white enough. Yet they overlook the fact that everyone needs to eat and have their clothes cleaned occasionally. Unless you are very wealthy and can pay for all of these services, it is in your best interest to develop at least basic proficiency. Having a home that runs smoothly can have a positive impact on every member of your family. In her book *The Time Bind* (1997), Arlie Hochschild observes, with some alarm, that many women she interviewed were working longer hours to avoid going home! A smoothly running home can even improve your willingness to be around members of your own family.

But there are other benefits. Let's think about your morning routine. Instead of frantically running around and looking for lost keys/schoolbooks/shoes, how would it be if everyone ate breakfast and calmly went out for the day? Do you think that this might influence the quality of your children's day? How about yours? A smoothly running home can do this.

Order also makes it easier, and more likely that your family will clean up after themselves. People are more apt to put things away when there is a place to put them, and if they don't have to fight with the contents of a drawer or cupboard every time they open it. Even young children can learn where to put things away if you clearly mark locations (such as drawers or shelves). And with that, we now move to my final suggestion—sharing the load.

Share the Load

You'll notice the title of this section is not "Getting Others to Help." That would imply that child and home care are your sole responsibility, and that others are "helping you out."

In most families, mothers do take on the majority of domestic work. Sometimes that is by conscious choice. You may be a mother at home, and you and your partner may have decided that it makes sense for you to handle things on the home front. That's great! If that is working for you, then by all means keep doing it. However, many times mothers do the majority of the domestic work because it is *assumed* that they should. This is where problems start, for it is not a fair arrangement. I believe that everyone who lives in your home should participate in its upkeep.

Trying to get others to participate does not happen overnight. I wish I could tell you some magic phrase that would make everyone want to pitch in right now. Of course, there is none. You probably already know two approaches that do not work: complaining and acting like a martyr.

You might wonder why you have to initiate this change. The most obvious reason is that your own behavior is all you have complete control over. Another is that if you've been doing most or all of the work, others have no stake in changing the status quo; change means more work for them. In this section, I describe three ways others can share the load, including your partner, your children, and outside help.

Chore Wars: The Gender Gap in Child and Home Care

As I noted previously, there are large differences in the amount of time men and women spend in domestic activities. Women at home full-time spend approximately fifty hours a week in child and home care. Employed women spend about thirty-five hours a week in these same activities. In contrast, men on average spend slightly less than eleven hours per week, with husbands of employed women spending approximately ten minutes extra per day and men with small children adding another ten minutes (Schwartz Cowan 1983). A recent commentary in *Business Week* indicates that this may have changed slightly, with men putting in around fourteen hours a week (Hammonds 1998).

The gender gap in housework is often fodder for comedians. Men, we're told, have an impaired cleaning gene. Their idea of "cleaning the bathroom" might include flushing the toilet and picking up a few things. But all kidding aside, the issue of who cleans the house and takes care of the kids is a major source of family strife. Relationships have ended over who takes out the garbage.

A recent survey in *Ladies' Home Journal* asked: "Given the chance to improve your husband, would you opt to make him a better lover, or would you rather he did more around the house?" Sixteen percent of respondents wanted a husband who performed better in bed. A full 46 percent wanted a husband who would "make the bed" (Johnson 2000).

Sometimes, men think that they *are* doing half the work. That's what Arlie Hochschild found in *The Second Shift* (1989). Men in her study thought that their responsibilities included taking care of the car, yard, and money, killing spiders, and barbecuing. Their wives' responsibilities were basically everything else. They honestly believed they were doing "half."

Schwartz Cowan (1983) makes a similar observation. Men's self-assigned jobs include taking out the trash, mowing the lawn, playing with the children, painting or fixing things, and occasionally shopping for household durables. Men typically do not do laundry, clean, or cook. They also frequently do not feed, clothe, bathe, or transport children. These tasks take a lot of time, and most of them are not "mommy-only," but can be shared with a partner.

Sometimes, lack of willingness to share chores reflects a deeper problem in the relationship. In this case, it's time to consider professional counseling. But the "chore wars" can become a major issue in any family. Below, I've listed some suggestions for seeking detente.

Recognize Expectations and Cognitive Distortions

When it comes to domestic work, everyone operates under assumptions that they probably aren't aware of. These assumptions include your sense of fairness, what you believe about men's versus women's work, your religious and cultural beliefs, and your memories of the way things were done in your family of origin. Not only do you probably have expectations about sex roles for various tasks, but you have ideas about the *way* things are done. You may honestly believe that *everyone* does a particular task the way you do, and that any other way is "stupid." Your partner may have the same beliefs about his approach. There may have been certain routines or rituals in your family of origin that you assumed were common to everyone. When your partner unwittingly violates one of these rules, you may then read too much into his behavior.

These issues may have come up before you had children. But they may be particularly salient now that you have children and the workload has dramatically increased, as Ron describes:

> The biggest roadblock Sarah and I ever hit was the difference in "styles" when doing chores. My mother-in-law did things differently than my mom. They weren't necessarily "wrong" or bad, but I did find them difficult to adjust to.

Sometimes issues like leaving the cap off the toothpaste are blown massively out of proportion because of our expectations. As I described in chapter 2, cognitive distortions can lead to a wide variety of problems. For example, a messy room may become "proof" that your partner does not care about you, or that he should know better. Kate describes her and her husband's different standards of cleanliness:

> Some things are important to me and not to him. He can sit and read on a bed where the sheets haven't been washed for three months. And he never buys shampoo; if we run out, he just uses soap.

Stefan, her husband, describes the household tasks he is responsible for:

> Kate would probably eat Cheerios every night, so usually I cook. If I crave pasta, I buy the stuff and make it (Johnson 2000).

It's important to be aware of situations when you might be influenced by cognitive distortions. For example, anytime you find yourself thinking or saying "never" or "always" (as in "he never helps"), it is a clue that you might be engaging in all-or-nothing thinking. When you are feeling more calm, ask yourself if it is really true that he *never* helps. Perhaps he doesn't help enough, but it is rarely helpful to discount the work that he is already doing.

Seek a Solution or Compromise

Sometimes you really do have different standards and are going to have to come to a compromise to bring peace to your home. Have a conversation about a particular issue when you are calm, and try to adopt a problem-solving approach. For example, if it drives you crazy when the lid is left off the toothpaste tube, can you get toothpaste that has a built-in lid? If dirty clothes on the bathroom floor are a problem, can you put a hamper in that room? If the dining room table gets covered with junk mail and other stuff, can you put a container near where your family comes into your home to collect these items? Try to be concrete about what is bothering each of you and what you each need. If you and your partner are clear about what your needs and expectations are, then you are in a better position to find a solution.

Corral the Mess

Corralling the mess is one strategy that can work well in areas that need compromise. Basically, you let someone be as messy as they want—within a confined space. For example, you may agree to not touch each other's home offices. You may request that he put clothes on a single chair in your room rather than on the floor. You may agree to keep the living room tidy most of the time, but let the family room have a more lived-in look. It's also helpful to have a container or drawer available in places where odds and ends accumulate, such as the kitchen, the entryway, or (in our house) the top of the stairs.

Beware the Witching Hour

Whether you are at home or employed outside it, one of the most challenging hours of the day is the hour before dinner. At-home moms often long for adult conversation after taking care of young children all day. Or they may yearn for some quiet time alone. Employed moms come home to mountains of chores, dinner that needs to be prepared, and homework that needs to be supervised. Partners returning from work at this time may also desperately want some time to decompress. Children are often at their most needy during this time as well. Efforts toward preventing family strife during the "witching hour" will pay big dividends. Every family must come up with a plan that works for them, but here are some possibilities.

If you are employed, you might find that it works well for you to sit and relax when you first get home. Even twenty minutes can help. Use this time to reconnect with your children or have some quiet time alone or with your partner. If you are an at-home mother, you might find it helpful to do most of the dinner preparations earlier in the day so that you will not be dealing with cranky children when you feel most frazzled. Have snacks ready to keep everyone from dissolving with hunger. Perhaps you can hire a teenager to help for a couple of hours, or trade dinner preparations with another mother. Think about keeping a stock of easy-to-prepare meals available so that others can pitch in. Be creative.

Getting Kids to Do Their Chores

It's important to involve children from a young age in caring for your home. Again, there is no magic formula here, but two of the best plans I've seen are in Stephen Covey's *The Seven Habits of Highly Effective People* (1989) and Don Aslett's *No Time to Clean* (2000). Both authors are fathers of large families and obviously speak from a wealth of experience. I will summarize their suggestions here, but if you would like additional information, I encourage you to read their books.

Teach by Example

Perhaps the best way to encourage kids to do their chores is through example. Instead of simply telling them to do something, offer to do it with them. Perhaps they are dawdling because they don't know what they are supposed to do. Maybe they are resisting because there is no place to put anything away. Or perhaps being sent to clean their rooms just seems too isolating and feels like a punishment. You could probably do kids' chores faster yourself, but in the long run, it is better to teach them to do the work themselves. And they are more likely to comply when doing chores means they have some one-on-one time with you or dad.

Make Chores Easy and Fun

Children are more likely to do chores if they are easy to do. Isn't this true for all of us? Making chores easy means having supplies they need at hand, and making sure they have a place to put things away. For young children, clearly indicate where they are supposed to put their possessions. Use pictures if they cannot yet read. Also make sure that they have a convenient trash can, one large enough that it doesn't tip over, and an accessible laundry hamper.

Consider whether any of the chores you want your child to do are too hard. For example, if you want your child to make his bed, ask yourself whether there are too many blankets and pillows. Is the bedspread heavy? Is the bed hard to get to because it is too close to the wall or other furniture? If you want him to put away his clothes, ask whether the bar in the closet is too high. Is it difficult for him to use hangers, and would pegs work better? Are the drawers clearly marked? (This is more important for younger children.) Is there a place for dirty clothes? Try to look at each job from your child's perspective.

Making chores easy for your child might also mean that you have to sort some possessions. I once read that by the time American children are five, they will have five times their body weight in toys. Most kids can part with some toys, especially those they have outgrown. When they are young, you'll probably need to do the sorting yourself, since young children rarely want to part with anything. As children mature, involve them in the act of giving to others who may not have as much. This is a wonderful opportunity for a life lesson. You might also consider letting them have a yard sale, from which they keep the proceeds. Your initial or periodic investment of time making chores easier for children will pay off with faster subsequent cleanups that the children can do themselves.

Finally think creatively about making each chore fun. One mother used to toss a handful of change in the dishwater each night. The child whose turn it was to wash dishes got to keep the change at the bottom of the sink. Her children could hardly wait until it was their turn to help with the dishes.

Let Them Experience the Consequences

Sometimes, children don't learn to take responsibility for their chores because their mothers bail them out. For example, mothers may continue to do their children's laundry even after they agree that their children should take this task over. If you let your children experience a day with no clean socks or underwear, they'll be more likely to make sure their laundry is done in the future (although some kids won't mind at all). This strategy especially works for older children or teens.

Counselor Kevin Leman (1987) describes the effective use of consequences in a case of a single mother and her teenage son and daughter. After a family meeting, mom and the teens agreed that the teens should start dinner each night. But she kept coming home night after night to kids on the phone or playing video games, and no dinner started. Her counselor then suggested that if dinner was not started when she returned home, she was to pick up her purse and go out to dinner—alone. There was adequate food in the house, so she knew her children would not starve. After three nights of this, her children got the message and started preparing dinner every night.

Some Mistakes We Make

Mothers can make it less likely that their children will participate in home care by their actions. For example, you may labor under the belief that you must do everything for your children. Sometimes this belief comes from your particular cultural or ethnic heritage, or the way that you were raised. Your mother may have done everything for you, so you try to emulate her. Conversely, your home life growing up may have been chaotic, so you do everything for your kids in an attempt to be different. Mothers at home may do it all because "what else do they have to do?" Employed mothers may do it all because they feel guilty about not being around more.

Some mothers think that it is bad for children to have to do chores. I propose an alternative view. Eventually, your children will leave your home. Are you doing them a service by letting them think that clean laundry appears in their drawers as if by magic? That food automatically appears in the cupboard? Won't they be better prepared for life if they know how to take care of themselves? If that doesn't persuade you, consider this: What do your actions tell your children about women if you are always the one who picks up after others?

Another common mistake mothers make is to be too critical of their children's efforts. If you did something, only to have someone come along and do it over, would it make you more or less likely to offer to help again? While it is nice to have "standards," you have to be careful with how you enforce them. This is your *home*, not Marine boot camp. If a job is not done to your satisfaction, see if you can figure out why. Perhaps you need to more fully explain what you want. Perhaps it is too hard to do. Remember that you have a dual focus when you ask a child to work around the house: getting the work done, and training the child.

Trading Money for Time: Paying for Help

This final suggestion can be a great adjunct to your work at home. My husband and I are avid do-it-yourselfers. Living in a house that is almost 200 years old gives us lots of opportunities to do things. But we have discovered that there are many times when it makes sense to pay someone else to do a job. Over the years, we have paid for services ranging from housecleaning to meal preparation to shopping to home improvement. We have also done all these things ourselves.

By purchasing services, you are trading money for time. Sometimes, paying for services can cost many times more than it would if you did the job yourself. But the cost can be equal or even less when the person providing the service has the equipment and/or the skill to do the job faster and better than you could. Make conscious choices about buying services, and you'll most likely find that doing so can really help in lightening your load.

Paying for help may involve either hiring a person or paying for a service that other people have provided. I would even include things like prepared food in this category, whether it is frozen, canned, or from a restaurant. During my most recent lupus flare, I learned to keep some prepared foods on hand for days when I am not feeling well. Although prepared foods are more expensive than those I could make myself, they are still substantially cheaper than going out to eat.

When considering whether to purchase a service, think not only about its cost, but about the time involved in acquiring the service. The time you save may not be significant if you must drive to drop off and pick up people or items. Similarly, if you must wait around for a person you hired, the time you save may be negligible. Consider also what your feelings are about the task. You or your partner may hate a task so much that you want to hire it out. Even if it costs more and doesn't save a lot of time, hiring a professional might be better than fighting about it or having to pay someone to fix a botched do-it-yourself job.

When we first moved into our old house, I was overwhelmed by the huge amount of painting that was needed. I decided to hire someone to do part of it, and the rest then seemed much more manageable. One of my friends is home with three small children. She has recently decided to pay someone to clean her house once a month since it is almost impossible for her to get any housework done during the day. I think it's a great idea! Here are some services you can purchase; new services are available all the time:

- Prepared foods

- Cleaning (maintenance or "big job")

- Child or elder care

- Boxing and shipping packages
- Yard care
- Laundry
- Pet care
- Personal shopping
- Home repair or maintenance
- Sewing
- Carpool
- Errands
- Clerical work
- Money services (banking, bookkeeping, paying bills, figuring taxes)
- Organization

What You Can Do

Throughout this chapter, I've offered specific suggestions to help you lighten your load at home. In closing, I'd like to offer a few more that will help you bring all this information together.

Start Small

If you have never tried to change your work at home before, you may find that you are overwhelmed by the information in this chapter. Don't be discouraged. Rome was not built in a day; it could take weeks or even months to get a good organization plan in place. As your needs change, you may find that you have to periodically update what you have done.

You can't do it all at once, but you can start by fixing one problem. It may take some time before things seem different for you, but every step you take moves you closer to your goal.

Be Flexible

As you think about dividing up some of your work, try not to think within the parameters of strict sex roles. For example, don't assume that handling money or home repair (or killing spiders) are jobs for men. You might be much better at these tasks than your partner. Along these lines, think about tasks that you like, are neutral about, or hate. You may have jobs you hate that your partner doesn't mind. A swap makes good sense. If you both hate a task, this might be a good one to hire out. Use talent and preference as your criteria rather than rules for who "should" be doing the task.

Take Time to Enjoy the Fruits of Your Labors

Sometimes, we start living *for* our homes rather than *in* them. With limited time and a crushing workload, this is easy to do. One of the reasons to lighten your load at home is to give you more time to spend with people you love. Make sure that you are not freeing up time just so you can do more work, but so you can enjoy yourself.

For Further Reading

A number of very helpful books on the market will help you lighten your load at home. Here are some favorites, organized by type. Happy reading!

Books about Making Your Home a More Inviting Place

These wonderful books all have great suggestions that cost little money.

Breathnach, S. B. 1995. *Simple Abundance: A Daybook of Comfort and Joy.* New York: Warner Books.

Moran, V. 1997. *Shelter for the Spirit.* New York: HarperPerennial.

Schaeffer, E. 1971. *The Hidden Art of Homemaking: Creative Ideas for Enriching Everyday Life.* Wheaton, Ill.: Tyndale House.

Stoddard, A. 1992. *Creating a Beautiful Home.* New York: Avon Books.

———. 1988. *Living a Beautiful Life: 500 Ways to Add Elegance, Order, Beauty and Joy to Every Day of Your Life.* New York: Morrow.

Resources for Household Organization

Both these books have excellent strategies for becoming more organized and thinking through the best solutions for you. And wait until you see this Web site!

Hemphill, B. 1998. *Taming the Paper Tiger at Home.* Washington, D.C.: Kiplinger Books.

Morgenstern, J. 1998. *Organizing from the Inside Out.* New York: Henry Holt and Company.

Organized Home: www.organizedhome.com

Resources for Streamlining Home Care

For helpful books on how to cut down on cleaning, Don Aslett is king. These books can save you hours. They are inspiring, funny, and very practical. He also has a mail-order cleaning-supply business (The Clean Report), and you can order his books from there too.

Aslett, D. 1984. *Clutter's Last Stand.* Cincinnati: Writer's Digest Books.

————. 1992. *Is There Life After Housework?* Cincinnati: Writer's Digest Books.

————. 2000. *No Time To Clean.* Pocatello, Ida.: Marsh Creek Press.

Aslett, D., and L. Aslett Simons. 1995. *Make Your House Do the Housework.* Cincinnati: Better Way Books.

Don Aslett's Clean Report: www.cleanreport.com

Resources for Involving Children in Home Care

These two books have great advice on involving children in the care of your home. Both are good reading in any case. These Web sites also have good information and products.

Aslett, D. 2000. *No Time to Clean.* Pocatello, Ida.: Marsh Creek Press.

Covey, S. R. 1989. *The Seven Habits of Highly Effective People.* New York: Fireside.

Chore Planner for Kids: purchase at www.magnaplanner.com

Christian Science Monitor: Return of Chores: Kids Meet Broom; search for "chores and kids" in the archive section of www.csmonitor.com

Tips for teaching responsibility: www.positivelearning.com=choretip.htm

CHAPTER 7

SO TIRED
MOTHERS AND FATIGUE

Fatigue is an excellent gauge of wellbeing because it is a very hard symptom to mask. The only way to get rid of fatigue is to treat the underlying causes. Fatigue has many faces, but they all say the same thing—the mental and physical load are too great. (Atkinson, *Women and Fatigue*, 1985, 6)

Fatigue is epidemic among women in general, and mothers in particular. Economist Juliet Schor, in her book *The Overworked American* (1992), describes how mothers talk to her about sleep the way someone who is starving talks about food. Fatigue can overshadow your life, making everything seem like too much trouble. If you find yourself dragging through your day, read on.

Eventually, lack of sleep has a negative effect on your health. But fatigue doesn't only affect you. People make mistakes when they are tired, and they are dangerous on the road. Lack of sleep can impact your ability to concentrate, handle stress, solve problems, and make decisions. You may become irritable with others and less productive (National Sleep Foundation 2000a).

Why Are Mothers So Tired?

Fatigue is common, but why are mothers so tired? In this section, I describe some of the factors that contribute to fatigue in mothers.

Overwork

Most obviously mothers are tired because they work so much. This can be true for mothers at home as well as those who are employed. In the classic *More Work for Mother* (1983), Ruth Schwartz Cowan writes that:

> With all her appliances and amenities, the status of being a "working mother" in the United States today is . . . virtually a guarantee of being overworked and perpetually exhausted. (213)

According to Schwartz Cowan, employed women typically work thirty-five hours per week in child and home care and forty hours per week in paid employment. That's seventy-five hours—a work week few sweatshops can match. And depending on the job, forty hours of paid work is probably conservative. It is easy to imagine a mother working eighty hours a week or more.

But as I mentioned in earlier chapters, employment outside the home is not the only activity that can make you feel fatigued. Overwork can also come from shouldering the burden of housework alone; caring for multiple children, children with health or behavioral concerns, or aging relatives; or doing some combination of these activities.

Not Enough Sleep

Another obvious source of fatigue is sleep deprivation, which is rampant in the United States. According to a recent survey by the National Sleep Foundation, most adults get less sleep than they need. On average, adults sleep a little less than seven hours per night, with a third of those surveyed indicating that they sleep less than six and a half hours per night. Forty-five percent said that they give up sleep to get more work done. With employed mothers putting in approximately seventy-five to eighty hours a week, it should come as no surprise to learn that they are skipping sleep. The National Sleep Foundation (2000b) describes it this way:

> Sleep problems have become a modern epidemic that is taking a catastrophic toll on our bodies and our minds . . . In our twenty-four-hour society, we steal nighttime hours for daytime activities, cheating ourselves of precious sleep. In the past century, we have reduced our average time asleep by 20 percent and in the past 25 years, added a month to our average annual work/commute time. Our

national sleep debt is on the rise. Our society has changed, but our bodies have not, and we are paying the price.

But staying up too late is not the only reason we don't get enough sleep. Below, I've summarized some of the most common reasons why people don't get the sleep that they need.

Insomnia

There are few things more frustrating than insomnia. You're lying awake in the middle of the night, watching the clock: 2 A.M., 3 A.M., 4 A.M. You realize that you have to be up in a couple of hours, but you've hardly slept at all. Morning comes too quickly and you will find yourself facing another day exhausted.

Shift Work

Shift work is notorious for causing sleep deprivation that results in daytime sleepiness. When someone works the night shift, she may try to sleep during the day. But this can be difficult. It's light outside and there is usually a lot more going on. Similarly, someone who works swing shift generally finishes work at 11 P.M. By the time she gets home and winds down, she may not get to sleep until 1 or 2 A.M. That doesn't leave much time to sleep if she needs to be up for the kids' morning routine.

On average, people who work shifts other than the day shift tend to sleep about four to six hours in a twenty-four-hour period. Mothers will often take swing or night shifts so they can be home with their children during the day. Some families find that this works well for them. But realize that it can be a major contributor to your fatigue. If you do decide to do shift work, it's best if you can stay on the same shift for at least three weeks. That's how long it takes the body to adjust.

Poor Sleeping Habits

Sometimes you don't get enough sleep because of bad sleep habits. Whereas these behaviors may not have caused a problem in the past, if you suddenly find that you are having difficulty getting the sleep you need, it might be helpful to take a look at your bedtime routine.

Some poor habits include drinking caffeinated beverages, exercising, or drinking alcohol too close to bedtime. Alcohol can make you feel drowsy, but it interferes with the quality of your sleep and can make you feel groggy in the morning. Other habits that can contribute to poor sleep include using your bed as your office or a place to watch TV.

Sleep Disorders

Two of the most common types of sleep disorders are obstructive sleep apnea and restless leg syndrome (RLS). Obstructive sleep apnea refers to a condition where the throat closes during sleep, and breathing is blocked. This causes people to waken many times throughout the night, making them very fatigued during the day. The person who suffers from this often snores loudly, also making it difficult for his or her partner to sleep well. Sufferers of RLS have the sensation that things are "crawling" under their skin whenever they lie down. They may find that their legs are in near-constant motion during the night. Not surprisingly, RLS also interrupts sleep and is often difficult for partners to endure.

Infant and Child Care

Caring for an infant or young child can keep you up at night. Young babies, in particular, need to wake frequently during the night to feed since their stomachs are so small. There is also increasing evidence that their neurological development is enhanced by having interactions with their mothers during the night. But this can be tough on you. The National Sleep Foundation poll (2000a) found that taking care of children disrupted sleep for 21 percent women compared with 12 percent of men. Even as children move past infancy, they still may be poor sleepers, and it is more often mothers who tend to their nighttime needs.

Bedmates

A partner's snoring can become a serious source of sleep disruption, and it is more likely to affect women. Twenty-two percent of women (versus 7 percent of men) reported that their partner's snoring interrupted their sleep (National Sleep Foundation 2000a). Moreover, women in a recent study who slept with a partner who snores had twenty-one brief awakenings per hour and spent only 74 percent of the night actually sleeping. These women were losing about sixty minutes of sleep per night (Health 2000).

You may have chosen to handle your children's nighttime needs by bringing them into bed with you. This can be a great solution that lets everyone sleep better. But you may find, at some point, that having children in your bed disrupts your sleep. This can be especially true with older children, who take up a lot more space. If you want your children near, you might consider having their bed next to yours, with each of you retaining your own bed space.

Along these same lines, you might find that your sleep is being disturbed by a pet. You may have a cat that gets social in the middle of the night or a dog that comes to nudge you awake at first light. If you are feeling fatigued much of the time, you may have to temporarily banish your pets from your bedroom.

Stress

Stress can make it hard to sleep, because, even when your body is resting, your overloaded mind is buzzing with what you need to do next. The National Sleep Foundation's 2000 poll found that 26 percent of women (compared with 16 percent of men) reported that stress interfered with their ability to sleep.

Depression

Fatigue is a symptom of depression, but it can also be a cause. Depression causes alterations in sleep. Particularly among people who are very depressed, sleep patterns differ compared with those who are not depressed. People who are depressed have REM sleep earlier in the night (see sidebar on normal sleep patterns). During REM sleep, the brain is in a highly active, almost awake state. This

WHAT IS NORMAL SLEEP?

Throughout the course of the night, we go through repeated cycles of sleep stages. We start in the lighter stages and move into deep sleep. Deep sleep is known as "slow wave sleep" (SWS), referring to the pattern of brain waves measured during these stages. After spending some time in slow wave sleep, we cycle back through the lighter stages, then go into REM sleep. REM is an acronym for "rapid eye movement." (In this stage of sleep a person's eyes often move even though they are closed.) It is during REM sleep that dreaming occurs. Also, during REM sleep, your brain shows patterns of activity similar to those you would see if you were awake.

As your night progresses, you start spending less time in SWS and more in REM. In normal sleep about 75 percent of your sleep time is non-REM, with the remaining 25 percent being REM.

earlier occurrence of REM may also explain one of the hallmark symptoms of depression, early-morning waking. Since the brain is so close to being awake during these times, it is easier to awaken. People who are depressed also spend less time in deep sleep. This contributes to not only fatigue but pain, since it is during deep sleep that muscles are repaired.

Post-Traumatic Stress Disorder (PTSD)

If you have suffered a major trauma or sustained a significant loss in your life, it may also be contributing to your insomnia. PTSD is notorious for causing sleep problems. The culprit seems to be intrusive thoughts, which can occur during the day or at night in the form of nightmares. Even if you don't have enough symptoms for a full-blown diagnosis of PTSD, you may still be experiencing intrusive thoughts.

One recent study found that intrusive thoughts were directly related to levels of norepinephrine: the higher the levels, the higher the rate of intrusive thoughts (Lemieux and Coe 1995). As you may recall, norepinephrine is one of the stress hormones. The traumatic event may have "flipped a switch" in your brain that has caused your body to be in a hyperaroused state. Consider using some mind-body techniques, such as relaxation training, to help counter the physiological reaction that the traumatic event created. You might find that as you process the trauma, your sleep improves.

Teresa describes how grief contributes to her almost daily feelings of exhaustion:

> We lost our first child, Miranda, when she was three months old. She had Down syndrome and died as a result of complications during heart surgery. We purposely conceived right away. Gwen was born a year and two weeks after Miranda. I had a difficult pregnancy with both, and between our bereavement, Gwen's intensely high needs, and my history of depression, I soon was quite depressed. When Gwen was seven months or so, I sought counseling and medication and eventually pulled out of it.
>
> Gwen's little brother Duncan is now one year old. I have not gone off the Zoloft yet. I made the difficult choice to remain on during the pregnancy and ever since. (Several attempts to go off had poor results.) I don't feel guilty about it, especially since he and I are doing ever so much better than Gwen and I did. However, it seems that sleep loss and exhaustion are my perpetual companions.

Underlying Physical Conditions

Fatigue can be the one and only sign of an underlying physical condition. The conditions with fatigue as a symptom are myriad and include anemia, hypothyroidism, diabetes, SAD, pregnancy, chronic fatigue syndrome, fibromyalgia, autoimmune diseases, and many others, even some cancers.

Iron-Deficiency Anemia

Anemia is one of the first conditions to consider as a cause of fatigue. It is remarkably common among women of childbearing age. Some 7.8 million women in America have iron deficiency and 3.3 million have iron-deficiency anemia. Iron deficiency can have a variety of causes. The most common is a diet lacking in iron, or a poor diet overall. Certain types of illnesses, especially those with chronic inflammation, can also cause iron-deficiency anemia. Anemia may also be due to bleeding from heavy menstrual periods, an ulcer, or, if you've recently had a baby, from a postpartum hemorrhage. Folic acid deficiency has also been linked to anemia. The symptoms of anemia are fatigue, pale or gray skin (including the linings of the eye and mouth), weakness, faintness, and breathlessness, and it can be diagnosed with a blood test.

Hypothyroidism

Hypothyroidism is another relatively common cause of fatigue in women. Thyroid hormone regulates our metabolism. Low levels can cause a wide range of symptoms, many of which are similar to those of depression. They include an inability to concentrate, tiredness, and forgetfulness. Low thyroid can also cause an intolerance to cold, persistently low body temperature, low blood pressure, weight gain, puffy face and eyes, constipation, and dry hair and skin.

Thyroid dysfunction can show up shortly after you've had a baby, and is one possible contributor to depression in new mothers. As you age, you are at increased risk for developing hypothyroidism. By age sixty, approximately 20 percent of women have low thyroid function. Hypothyroidism also is common in people with chronic fatigue syndrome, fibromyalgia, and some autoimmune diseases. For example, Teitelbaum (1996) describes how almost half of his chronic fatigue patients are also hypothyroid. Women with one or more of these conditions tend to experience a double or even triple whammy of fatigue.

Diabetes

Diabetes can cause significant levels of fatigue, and many with diabetes do not even realize that they have it. Other symptoms can include frequent urination, thirst, blurry vision, weight loss, and hunger, but fatigue may be your one and only symptom. Diabetes is diagnosed with a blood test.

Seasonal Affective Disorder (SAD)

Seasonal affective disorder (SAD) is a type of depression that occurs when there is less light available, such as during the winter. You may not experience SAD as depression per se, but you may notice a lack of energy in the winter. If you live in a part of the country with short winter days, or where it rains a lot and is frequently overcast, you may have SAD without realizing it. Are you more energetic in the spring and summer? During the winter, do you find that you sleep more and crave foods loaded with carbohydrates? Do you tend to pack on an extra ten to twenty pounds during the winter, and easily lose it when the days start getting longer? Any of these might indicate SAD, which is easily remedied with light therapy.

Pregnancy

We don't often think of pregnancy as a contributor to fatigue, but fatigue is common in both early and late pregnancy. And the more children you already have, the more likely you are to be fatigued during subsequent pregnancies. During a first pregnancy, you may have had plenty of time to rest when you felt tired, or to nap during the day. This becomes much more difficult when you already have children at home. Recovery from birth may also be more challenging if you are coming home to other children. Like many American mothers, you might find yourself alone after a few days, not only to recover, but also to care for your other children.

Chronic Fatigue Syndrome

Chronic fatigue syndrome (CFS) first made its appearance a few years ago as an official diagnosis. However, the phenomenon has been observed for many years. CFS refers to a constellation of symptoms that include low-grade fevers, persistent infections, sore throat, headaches, pains in muscles and joints, and tender lymph nodes. But the hallmark symptom is overwhelming fatigue that worsens with activity. Depression and anxiety are both common in those with CFS.

CFS often starts with an infection or illness that doesn't seem to get better. Diagnosis of this condition is tricky since there are no laboratory tests that confirm its existence (although the presence of the Epstein-Barr virus has been noted in some sufferers). Doctors typically make the diagnosis by eliminating other illnesses that could be causing the fatigue.

As with many other types of chronic illness, current stressors can trigger a relapse of CFS symptoms. Rose, who was diagnosed with CFS several years ago, saw her symptoms return with a vengeance after her husband was diagnosed with cancer. She also had two young children still at home, one of whom had Down syndrome.

CFS is still a controversial diagnosis. It has been called the "yuppie flu" by those who doubt whether it really exists. Public skepticism makes those who suffer from it feel bad, and it reinforces their belief that no one understands what they are going through. But researchers in the field feel that once its cause is officially documented, many people will hang their heads in shame over the way CFS sufferers have been treated.

Fibromyalgia

Fibromyalgia (FM) is also a fairly new diagnosis and has many similarities to CFS. FM is a condition that causes diffuse soft tissue pain. Fatigue is another hallmark symptom. The people who suffer from it are overwhelmingly women, causing some to dismiss its legitimacy. Another problem is that there are no laboratory tests that can confirm the diagnosis. Diagnosis is made by pressing "tender points" at various places in the body. These locations are not tender among the general population, but are very painful for those who suffer from FM. Diagnosis is usually made by a rheumatologist, a physician who specializes in the treatment of arthritis and other rheumatic diseases. Although FM is not technically a form of arthritis, rheumatologists who developed the diagnostic criteria and have been at the forefront in studying this condition. FM also tends to co-occur with certain types of inflammatory arthritis, such as rheumatoid arthritis and lupus.

Women suffering from FM can often point to a traumatic event that led to the onset of their symptoms, such as a car accident, a rape, or armed robbery. Many of these women have family members who had similar conditions, indicating that there may be a genetic predisposition to FM.

FM seems to do something to sleep patterns. During slow wave sleep, alpha waves (which characterize an awake brain) intrude, causing FM patients to not get sufficient slow wave sleep. The body needs slow wave sleep to repair the "microtrauma" to muscles that occurs throughout the day. If this repair process is interrupted, the result is overall muscle pain. Researchers have even been able to induce this in the laboratory. Whenever healthy volunteers went into deep sleep, the lab technicians would wake them up. After a night of this type of interrupted sleep, the patients in the study reported over-all body pain.

Fibromyalgia also tends to perpetuate both fatigue and pain because of muscle deconditioning. When you are exhausted, the last thing you want to do is exercise; or, without meaning to, you can exercise too much, have a dramatic increase in pain for a week or more, and stop exercising. In either case lack of exercise may contribute to deconditioning of muscles, which leads to more fatigue in the future.

Autoimmune Diseases

Statistically, autoimmune diseases are fairly rare. However, I have included them because women of childbearing age are particularly vulnerable to many autoimmune diseases, and they experience overwhelming fatigue as a result. Autoimmunity is the process by which the body loses its ability to distinguish "self" from "not self," and your immune system attacks your organs as it would an outside invader.

Autoimmune diseases include the 150 forms of inflammatory arthritis, two of the most common of which are rheumatoid arthritis and systemic lupus erythermatosus. Other less common diseases include sarcoidosis and scleroderma. Multiple sclerosis, while not a form of arthritis, is another autoimmune disease that strikes women of childbearing age. Women may have their first significant episode of an autoimmune disease while pregnant or shortly after giving birth. These illnesses can also cause multiple miscarriages and infertility.

A recent article in the journal *Arthritis & Rheumatism* indicated that hormones associated with breastfeeding can trigger a flare of rheumatoid arthritis or other forms of inflammatory arthritis (Barrett et al. 2000). The authors speculated that the hormone prolactin was to blame. Surgery can also trigger an episode, so mothers who have had a cesarean section are at increased risk. Finally, sleep deprivation can trigger an episode.

Not only do autoimmune diseases contribute to fatigue, but some treatments can as well. Prednisone and other corticosteroids are frequent treatments for autoimmune disease, especially during periods of disease activity. Prednisone can not only lead to rapid weight gain, but it can also cause muscle wasting. The lack of muscle tone and the additional weight can both contribute to a lack of energy. Patients who have been on steroids for any length of time may also find that they are susceptible to recurring yeast infections. "Yeast overgrowth" is a controversial diagnosis, yet practitioners of alternative medicine have recognized its contribution to chronic fatigue for many years (Goldberg 1998).

Fatigue can also trigger a flare of symptoms. The body perceives that you are under attack when you are sleep-deprived. Therefore, at the first sign of sleep deprivation, it fires up the immune system. People with autoimmune diseases already have an immune system that is too active, so sleep deprivation can increase their sympotoms.

What You Can Do

Fortunately, there are many positive steps you can take to help alleviate some of the fatigue you feel. While you may not eliminate fatigue, you no longer have to consider overwhelming tiredness as a way of life.

Determine Your Sleep Needs

Often, we feel we are getting enough sleep when we really aren't. So how can you tell?

- Do you need an alarm clock to wake you every morning?

- Do you roll over in the morning and "catch a few more z's"?

- Do you try to catch up on your sleep over the weekend?

- Do you feel drowsy after a big meal, in an overheated room, or during a long meeting?

If you are getting enough sleep, the answer to each of these questions should be "no" (National Sleep Foundation 2000b). To determine how much you need, try this on your next vacation. Go to bed when you are tired, and get up when you are finished sleeping. For the first few days, you may need to get rid of your accumulated sleep debt. After that, you will have a pretty good idea of how much sleep you need to feel restored.

Practice Good Sleep Hygiene

When you are having sleep problems, it's time to consider activities that might be interfering with your sleep.

First establish good bedtime rituals. Before bedtime, allow yourself some time to wind down. Try not to eat anything that is heavy or will upset your stomach at least two hours before bedtime. Also avoid caffeine and more than one alcoholic drink in the evenings, and do not exercise in the two or three hours before bed. Exercise tends to rev you up, making it difficult for you to sleep.

Get out of the habit of doing anything in your bed but sleeping and having sex. Often, people who suffer from insomnia spend nonsleeping time on or in their beds, watching TV, reading, catching up on work. If you are having sleep problems, it's time to stop this behavior, at least for now. When you have insomnia, get out of bed and do something boring. When you are feeling sleepy, try sleeping again. You want to associate "bed" with "sleep"; lying there wide awake gives you the opposite association. Similarly, bed will lose its sleep association if it becomes an extension of your office.

Make the Bedroom Pleasant

If you are having trouble sleeping, it's important that your bedroom be an oasis of physical and psychological comfort and calm. Since your bedroom is private, it may be the part of your home you ignore. Sometimes, all the clutter in your house ends up in your room.

Your bedroom should be a comfortable temperature, neither too hot nor too cold. If your mattress feels too hard, consider getting an "egg-crate" foam cushion. Also, find a pillow that gives good support without putting a kink in your neck. Pay attention to anything you feel might be keeping you from sleeping. Are you sleeping in something comfortable? Do your legs get tangled in the sheets? Normally, you might be able to ignore these little annoyances, but when you are having trouble sleeping, you must consider them all.

If your bedroom is facing a noisy street, or is next to noisy neighbors, consider getting a white noise machine or portable stereo to block some of these sounds. If the moon or streetlights shine in your face at night, use shades or reposition your bed to keep the light from disturbing your sleep.

Try not to have a home office in your bedroom. If it's unavoidable, cover your desk at night when you are not working. You might also find it stressful to have an end table overflowing with books and magazines you never get to, reminding you of work that you never seem to have time to finish. If you are having sleep troubles, stash your mound of reading materials out of sight.

Take Care of Your Body

You knew I would say this. As I've said elsewhere, we need to eat well, exercise, drink enough water, and reduce our stress. But this is often easier said than done.

Diet

The current barrage of information on diet is very confusing. Should we eat a high protein or a high carbohydrates diet ? Proponents of both approaches think theirs is best and that the other will *kill* you.

So what are you supposed to do? I've come to a few of conclusions.

First, humans are pretty flexible. We can live well on protein or carbohydrates. The safest approach is probably somewhere in the middle. Eat carbohydrates, but mostly the unrefined kind found in whole grains, fruits and vegetables, and legumes. Drink plenty of water and eat an adequate amount of protein. You may have to experiment, especially with the amount of protein, to find out what works best for you.

Second, what works well for you doesn't necessarily work well for your neighbor. Everyone has different eating histories, food sensitivities, and likes. You should honor those.

Third, eat food that tastes good and is of good quality. If you are going to have chocolate, have a small portion of quality chocolate. If you want a baked treat, have a piece of cake that you made yourself or got at a bakery rather than some fat-free concoction that was baked two weeks ago.

Something else to consider with regard to carbohydrates and protein is timing. Protein gives you sustained energy, whereas carbohydrates can make you groggy. So carbohydrates might be more appropriate for an evening meal and protein better for the afternoon. Again, experiment and see what works best for you.

Exercise

In addition to watching your diet, you also need to exercise. I know that when you are tired, this is the last thing you feel like doing. But exercise is energizing.

If you haven't been exercising start small, with five minutes per day of walking or strength training with light weights. Gradually increase this time as you feel able. Being creative about when and where you exercise can help you add exercise to your day in a natural way so it doesn't feel like one more item that you "have to" do. While you're standing at the kitchen sink or talking on the phone, you can do calf raises. While you are watching TV, you can use some exercise equipment. You can use lunch hours at work, even if you have only ten extra minutes, to take a brisk walk. Exercise is one of the single most powerful things we can do to help ourselves. Be sure to make time for it.

If you have CFS, FM, or an autoimmune disease, you may need the assistance of your physical therapist. Take things slowly so that you don't overdo. You might also consider a program of gentle strength training to rebuild muscles that have wasted due to lack of use or medications.

Rest

A brief nap can be restorative so think creatively about ways you can get some rest during the day. If you've been up caring for a child at night, do whatever you can to be able to rest during the day. If at all possible, rest when your child rests. Don't use this time to catch up on chores. Napping may also mean that other things don't get done—and that can be okay. Consider delegating these tasks or eliminating them from your list.

Even if you are employed, you might be able to squeeze rest into your day. Companies are beginning to realize that workers who nap are more productive and have fewer accidents at work. Investigate the possibility.

One caution about napping: Don't sleep too long or too close to your normal bedtime. This can interfere with your regular night's sleep.

Make Necessary Accommodations

If you have a chronic condition, you may have an ongoing battle with fatigue even after the condition has been identified and treated. You might need to exercise, but in a limited way. You might also need to limit other activities to conserve your energy.

In a presentation at the 1999 American College of Rheumatology meetings in Boston, rheumatologist David Isenberg reported on his findings for lupus patients in his practice. He asked his patients to describe their worst symptom, fully expecting them to say "fear of death," or "facial disfigurement." He was quite surprised to learn that his patients considered fatigue to be their worst symptom. His findings underscore one of the major challenges that mothers with chronic conditions face.

Ellen describes how she made accommodations for the physical disability that often left her very tired. She decided to quit her job so that she could have more control over her schedule:

> Being a teacher was wonderful, but I loved being home with our three boys. It was good for me emotionally and physically not to have the pressures of a job. I had polio when I was a child, and wore a brace or used crutches. I was able to do just about anything I wanted, but found stress was hard on me. Being in charge of my day with the boys made it easier to keep my activities in line. I did less and less as the boys grew, since even getting into their school required more energy than I had, and I resisted getting a wheelchair or scooter for assistance.
>
> Years later, I found out that I had new physical problems from having had polio: my nerves and muscles are wearing out. I had to quit my job with the health department as a breastfeeding and nutrition educator. This led to sleeping a lot and depression. But I keep active on the computer writing a nutrition column for polio survivors with post polio syndrome (PPS). My Web site helps me keep in touch with and help others who are discovering that PPS is affecting their health and lives in new ways, too. This feels good. My entire family is so supportive, and that is so very helpful to me as I face new health problems.
>
> I'm just trying to take one day at a time, and enjoying each one to the fullest. I'm resting a lot, but not giving up in any way! We just spent a month in Europe traveling by train. We planned it so I could rest, and we took a scooter to ride since I can't walk too far. I was able to see Rome "on foot," and to visit our oldest son and his wife in Sicily. They are expecting a baby in May: our first grandchild. Life is good!

If you have a physical disability but don't already have a handicapped tag for your car you might consider getting one. I originally got one so I could limit my sun exposure (which can trigger a lupus flare). But I was absolutely amazed at the difference it made in my fatigue level.

Should You See a Doctor?

Fatigue is a very common complaint in primary care practice. Though it can be challenging for a doctor to track down its source, consulting a doctor may be a good idea if one or more of the following is true:

- The fatigue has lasted for more than three weeks.
- It is getting worse.
- It is interfering with your work, or your relationships with your family.

When you see a doctor, request a complete blood count (CBC). This will tell your doctor if you are anemic or have too much iron in your system. If you had a postpartum hemorrhage within the past year, your blood iron levels may be low. A CBC will also indicate if you have an infection. You might also request thyroid and glucose tests. If you have a family history of autoimmune disease, or have some other symptoms, such as joint pain, low-grade fevers, or frequent infections you might also consider requesting a sedimentation or "sed" rate. This is a general measure of inflammation. An elevated sed rate can indicate infection, autoimmune disease, and even cancer, and may cue your doctor to look further into the source of your fatigue.

You may have been the medical route and not been satisfied. Another option is to consider herbal remedies that will help you sleep. Consult with a naturopath or physician trained in herbal medicine. With sedating herbs, it's best that you not try to treat yourself. Also, be sure to tell your regular doctor about any herbs that you plan to take, since these can interact with other medications you may already be taking.

Be Creative with Sleeping Arrangements

Americans, in particular, have pretty rigid ideas about where people should sleep. Parents are encouraged to keep children out of their room. Partners are encouraged to always sleep in the same room. If your current sleeping arrangements are working for you, by all means, leave them alone! But if you are chronically fatigued, it may be time to put some of these "shoulds" aside—at least for the time being.

For example, you and your child (or children) might sleep better if you are in the same room. In many countries of the world, including industrialized countries like Japan, mothers and babies sleep together. This is called "cosleeping." You might consider having your baby in bed with you, or if this is not comfortable, you might try having your baby or child beside your bed in a bassinet, crib, or youth bed. (The list at the end of this chapter has resources for safe cosleeping).

A trickier issue is what to do about a snoring partner, or one whose other sleep disorders keep you awake. The first approach is to talk to your partner about how his snoring is impacting you. Be extra careful here, since this is not something he's doing deliberately. Try to frame this as a couple's problem that you want to find a solution for. Snoring may improve if your partner tries different positions for sleeping. Your partner can be checked for sleep apnea, and there may be an appliance that can help. There may also be medication that will help with problems like restless leg movements. You can try things, too, including earplugs, sleeping in a different room or bed. You may find that an occasional night apart makes all the difference in how you feel the next morning. You may want to save this for a last resort. It can be hard for your partner not to take this as a rejection, so approach the subject carefully.

Conclusion

Daily fatigue is something many mothers experience. Fortunately, you don't have to walk through every day feeling like one of the living dead. Getting enough good-quality sleep may be just what you need to face some of the other challenges you meet during your time as a mother, and there are steps you can take to get it.

For Further Reading

Many available books are helpful in identifying the multiple causes of fatigue. I've listed some of the better ones I've found below, along with some good Web sites

Resources for Fatigue in General

Atkinson, H. 1985. *Women and Fatigue*. New York: Pocket Books.

Ford, N. 2000. *How to Get a Good Night's Sleep: 75 Natural Sleep Prescriptions*. New York: Barnes & Noble Books.

Monson, N. 1999. *Smart Guide to Boosting Your Energy*. New York: John Wiley and Sons.

Natelson, B. H. 1998. *Facing and Fighting Fatigue: A Practical Approach.* New Haven, Conn.: Yale University Press.

Smith, P. 1999. *The Energy Edge: Ten Simple Strategies to Soar Past Fatigue, Boost Energy, Shed Stress, and Reclaim Your Life.* New York: HarperInformation.

Wade, C. 2000. *Natural Energy Boosters.* New York: Barnes & Noble Books.

American Wholehealth Inc.: Go to "health topics" in the wholehealth library at www.americanwholehealth.com

Prevention: Go to Health Tools, Vitamin Dispenser, then Fatigue at www.healthyideas.com

Resources for Specific Conditions

Conly, E. J. 1998. *America Exhausted: Breakthrough Treatment on Fatigue and Fibromyalgia.* Flint, Mich.: Vitality Press.

Dement, W. C., and C. Vaughan. 2000. *The Promise of Sleep: A Pioneer of Sleep Medicine Explores the Vital Connection Between Health, Happiness, and a Good Night's Sleep.* New York: Dell Publishing.

Friedberg, F. 1995. *Coping with Chronic Fatigue Syndrome.* Oakland, Calif.: New Harbinger.

Goldberg, B. 1998. *Chronic Fatigue, Fibromyalgia, and Environmental Illness: 26 Doctors Show You How They Reverse These Conditions with Clinically Proven Alternative Therapies.* Tiburon, Calif.: Future Medicine Press.

Rosenthal, N. E. 1998. *Winter Blues: Seasonal Affective Disorder. What It Is and How to Overcome It.* New York: The Guilford Press.

Smyth, A., and W. C. Thompson. 1990. *Seasonal Affective Disorder: Winter Depression. Who Gets it? What Causes It? And How to Cure It?* London: Thorsons.

Starlanyl, D. J., and M. E. Copeland. 1996. *Fibromyalgia & Chronic Myofascial Pain Syndrome: A Survival Manual.* Oakland, Calif.: New Harbinger.

Teitelbaum, J. 1996. *From Fatigued to Fantastic.* Garden City Park, New York: Avery.

Sleep Disorders

National Center on Sleep Disorders Research, at National Heart, Lung, and Blood Institute: www.nhlbi.nih.gov

National Sleep Foundation: www.sleepfoundation.org

Chronic Fatigue Syndrome

American Association for Chronic Fatigue Syndrome: www.aacfs.org

The CFIDS Association of America: www.cfids.org

Mediconsult: Pick "chronic fatigue syndrome" at www. mediconsult.com

Fibromyalgia

Fibromyalgia and Chronic Myofascial Pain Syndrome: www.sover.net /~devstar/

Fibromyalgia Files: www.geocities.com/cfsdays/fmsfiles.htm

Healthtouch: search for "fibromyalgia" at www.healthtouch.com
USA Fibromyalgia Association: www.w2.com/fibro1.html

Seasonal Affective Disorder

Columbia University: Search for "light therapy in winter": www.colum-
bia.edu
Outside In: www.outsidein.co.uk
Seasonal Light and SAD Homepage: www.geocities.com/lpuls.geo
/sadhome.html
The Sunbox Company: www.sunbox.com

Other Conditions

American Academy of Allergy, Asthma, and Immunology: www.aaaai.org
American Thyroid Association: www.thyroid.org

Resources for Child/Infant Sleep Problems/Safe Cosleeping

It's important to avoid cosleeping under certain conditions (e.g., while on medication that makes you drowsy). But safe cosleeping occurs all over the world. If you want to give cosleeping a try, look at these resources.

Sears, W. 1999. *Nighttime Parenting: How to Get Your Baby and Child to Sleep.* New York: Dutton/Plume.
Thevenin, T. 1987. *The Family Bed: An Age-old Concept in Child Rearing.* Garden City Park, N.Y.: Avery.
La Leche League International: www.lalecheleague.org
Online: Nurturing www.nurturing.ca
Parentingweb: Click on Attachment Parenting at www. parentingweb.com

CHAPTER 8

THE LONG SHADOW
ADULT SURVIVORS OF CHILDHOOD ABUSE

References to "the dysfunctional family" are so common these days they are almost a cliché. But behind the cliché is the sad reality: some families are poisonous for children. Childhood abuse, particularly when severe, can cast a long shadow over your life, influencing your emotional state and how you relate to others. Even when not abusive, families can be dysfunctional in other ways, such as having a chronically depressed, mentally ill, or substance-abusing parent. Your upbringing may have left you poorly equipped to parent your own children. In this chapter, I describe how experiences of some of the most common types of abuse and family dysfunction could be affecting you, and suggest some ways you can seek healing.

Types of Childhood Abuse and Trauma

Child abuse takes a wide variety of forms, and can range from mild to severe. Even competent parents make mistakes and have difficulties. Abuse can occur both inside the family and with people who are not family members. By and large, however, the experiences I am describing occur within the home. In severely dysfunctional homes, it's not unusual for several types of abuse to occur at the same time. For example, someone who is sexually abusive is often physically abusive as well. In families where there is partner abuse, there is also likely to be parental depression and substance abuse. The overall level of severity and degree of family pathology is what seems to most affect children exposed to any of these types of abuse.

Sexual Abuse

One of the most highly studied forms of abuse is child sexual abuse. Experiences can include everything from fondling to oral, vaginal, or anal penetration. And girls are likelier to experience sexual abuse than boys (Sedlak and Broadhurst 1996). Approximately 20 percent of women (1 in 5), and 5 to 10 percent of men (1 in 10 to 20) have been sexually abused as children. The peak age of vulnerability is between seven and thirteen years of age, but children older and much younger have been abused (Finkelhor 1994).

Why does sexual abuse happen more to girls? Two possible reasons have been offered, but neither completely explains sexual abuse. One explanation is male dominance of women. In this framework, men are described as the abusers of women and girls, especially within the family. Research has in fact demonstrated that sexual abusers are overwhelmingly male, and the majority of victims are female. But this does not explain all sexual abuse. There are male victims and female perpetrators too.

Access is another possible explanation for the sex difference in sexual abuse rates. Girls are most likely to be abused by family members, especially stepfathers, while boys are more likely to be abused outside the family. Girls may be more vulnerable to sexual abuse because the people most likely to abuse them are right in their homes. For girls, approximately half of perpetrators are family members; for boys only 10 to 20 percent are. While fathers and stepfathers are the most likely to abuse, other family members can also be abusive, including brothers, uncles, grandfathers, and "friends of the family."

Mothers and other female relatives can also be sexually abusive. So far, we know little about female perpetrators. Some believe that this is because it is rare to be sexually abused by a mother. Others, however, including some adult survivors who were molested by their mothers, believe that female perpetration is the most secretive and closeted of all types of sexual abuse.

Physical Abuse

We know more about sexual abuse, but physical abuse is actually more common. However, unlike with sexual abuse, boys and girls are equally likely to be physically abused (Sedlak and Broadhurst

1996). Physical abuse ranges from spanking that "crosses the line" (and people are still arguing about where that line is) to torture and even murder.

Children are most vulnerable to physical abuse in the first three years of life, but it can occur at any time. When children are young, mothers are most likely to be the abusers. But any family member can be abusive. And as I describe in the next two chapters, children who have difficult temperaments or disabilities, especially ones that make them challenging to care for, are at higher risk for physical abuse (Sullivan and Knutson 2000).

Recently, researchers have become interested in physical abuse among siblings. Sibling physical abuse is one of the most common forms of family violence. In most families, it is relatively mild. Because it occurs frequently, we tend to think of it as "normal." But sibling abuse can be very severe and have many of the same consequences as parental abuse. In interviewing adult survivors of child sexual abuse, I have found that abuse by a brother or sister was often brutal and sadistic. (This seemed especially true when there was a substantial age difference.) I wouldn't be at all surprised to find something similar with regard to physical abuse.

Sibling abuse, especially in its more severe forms, often reflects an overall level of family pathology. Chances are, there are other types of maltreatment present as well. Parents may be abusive, or at the very least, neglectful. Not surprisingly, having multiple abusers makes the overall abuse experience more severe.

Neglect

Neglect is by far the most common type of child maltreatment. Unlike physical or sexual abuse, where something is actually *done*, neglect involves *failure to do* something. Types of neglect include not providing food, clothing, or medical attention, as well as failure to supervise or provide a safe environment or proper education. (Unfortunately, families who home-school are often harassed under the education portion of the neglect laws.)

Not surprisingly, families who neglect their children are often chaotic. And while poverty accounts for some neglect, there usually is something else going on, especially in chronically neglectful homes. For example, Beth's mother and father were both alcoholics. She was frequently hungry because her parents spent the money they had on alcohol. In a paper entitled "The Psychological Ecology of the Neglectful Mother," (1985) Norman Polansky and his colleagues gathered a group of mothers identified as "neglectful" by social services. They then found another group of mothers who were not neglectful, but had the same income level, education, marital status, ethnicity, and even neighborhood as the neglectful mothers. What they found was illuminating. The mothers identified as neglectful were depressed, had few friends, and seemed unable to take advantage of resources that were available to them in their communities.

Depression in mothers and fathers is also related to neglect. Recall from chapter 2 that depression influences a mother's ability to interact with her children. One interaction style of depressed mothers is "avoidant." Avoidant mothers disengage from their children, and ignore them much of the time. The other style, "angry-intrusive," is a risk factor for physical abuse (I'll discuss this in a minute).

Neglect in more affluent families may happen in more subtle forms. Food and clothing may be provided, but the parents might be emotionally absent, showing little interest in their children. Mothers or fathers may have been so emotionally immature that their children had to care for them, rather than the other way around. Parents can also be so uninvolved that they fail to notice when something really serious occurs in their children's lives. Both Marilyn and Sandy were raised in middle-class homes with neglectful, substance-abusing mothers. Both were raped as teens by kids from their schools. Neither girl's family noticed the abrupt change in her behavior after she was raped. These families never asked why their daughters were acting so strangely.

Emotional and Verbal Abuse

In recent years, a public service campaign reminded us that "words can hit as hard as a fist." For many people, emotional abuse is the worst type of maltreatment. Emotional and verbal abuse can take a variety of forms. It can involve name-calling and saying hateful things. It can include constant comparisons between siblings, or calling a child "stupid," or "fat," or "ugly," or "a loser." It can consist of mocking or holding a child up to shame, embarrassing her in front of her friends or even strangers. It can also include abandonment or threat of abandonment. Especially for young children, having a parent threaten to leave them someplace can be highly traumatizing. Any of these experiences can be the source of many of the negative internal messages that replay in your mind.

Emotional and verbal abuse often accompanies other forms of family violence and child maltreatment. Some adult survivors recount how their mothers or fathers made them feel responsible for the abuse that was inflicted upon them. It can be especially devastating when girls are told that they are responsible for "seducing" someone who sexually abuses them. These children often end up in abusive relationships as adults—perhaps with abusers who also blame their victims for the abuse: "If you would just keep the house clean, I wouldn't have to do this." Women in abusive adult relationships may have internalized these messages to such an extent that they stay, since "no one else would want me."

Unfortunately, many forms of emotional abuse also pass for "humor" in a family. Some parents find saying degrading things to be funny. Even some so-called family movies have very ugly examples of verbal and emotional abuse (the opening scenes of the movie *Home Alone* are an example). Sometimes, this type of abuse is perpetrated by parents. Other times, it is brothers and sisters. In most families, siblings will name-call and tease. But as parents, we can either tolerate it or not.

A particularly heinous form of emotional abuse is when the abusive parent or sibling hits, tortures, or kills a child's beloved pet. Researcher Frank Ascione of Utah State University has done groundbreaking research in this area (Ascione 1995). In talking to women in battered women's shelters, he found that women often stayed in battering relationships because they feared for the life of a beloved cat or dog. When a pet was killed, it was often this event that made the woman finally leave. And finally, he found that for women and children, watching their pets suffer was one of the most traumatic aspects of their entire abuse experiences.

Parental Substance Abuse or Mental Illness

Families where there is substance abuse or mental illness bring many pressures to bear on their children. Children of alcoholics or substance abusers, especially the oldest girl, often find that they are the "little adults" in the family. If your parents were substance abusers, you may have been responsible for meeting your parents' emotional needs rather than the other way around. You may have also had to provide for the other children in the family, being the one who made sure that there was food in the house and that your brothers and sisters had adequate clothing and did their homework after school. You might find that you are still taking care of lots of other people, and that it's never reciprocal. Not surprisingly, parental substance abuse can increase the risk for physical or sexual abuse as well. This is not to say that alcohol or drugs *cause* parents to abuse.

But they can lower inhibitions and allow behaviors that might not have occurred in a sober state.

Depression and other mental illnesses can increase not only the risk of neglect but also of physical abuse. Recall that one interaction style that depressed mothers exhibit is angry-intrusive. The interactions these depressed mothers have with their children tend to be hostile, and the mothers themselves exhibit a lot of anger, perhaps crossing a line and physically abusing a child.

Substance abuse and mental illness are also related to parents' failure to protect children. A parent who is often high, drunk, or incapacitated may not be able to adequately keep children safe. They may bring people to their homes who abuse their children. Substance-abusing parents may also provide their children an early introduction to alcohol or drugs, either by having them easily available, or even by encouraging their use.

Children Witnessing Domestic Violence

Children who have watched a parent, usually their mother, being beaten often show many signs of disturbance, even if they themselves were never actually abused. Catherine Koverola of the University of Maryland, Baltimore recently found that children who had witnessed their mothers being beaten were distressed, poorly adjusted, and showed signs of trauma that were the same, or even worse, than children who had been sexually abused (Koverola and Morohan 2000). In the case of domestic abuse, staying together "for the sake of the children" is a disastrous idea.

The kinds of domestic violence that children witness range from fairly mild to very severe. Some children have even witnessed their fathers killing their mothers. Child witnessing also tends to co-occur with other forms of maltreatment. For example, abusive partners may also abuse their children. Substance abuse and mental illness may afflict the abuser, and depression in abused partners and children is particularly likely. Children witnessing domestic abuse also often experience family violence as adults. I know one particularly pathological family, in which all four children witnessed their mother being beaten. The two boys grew up to beat their wives, and the two girls both married or lived with a series of abusive men. As the parents got older, the children would, on occasion, hit them too. Not surprisingly, both parents and all four children were substance abusers as well.

Prolonged Separation, or Parent Illness or Death

Difficulties in childhood may also have nothing to do with family dysfunction per se, but may be due to a child's prolonged separation from her parents. The effects on you of political strife, natural disaster, illness, or death are similar to those experienced by people who suffered abuse within their families.

If you were ill as a child, you may have been separated from your family and forced to undergo invasive and painful procedures. Children who have had multiple hospitalizations are at increased risk for depression and traumatic-stress reactions. We're now realizing that even adults who endure painful medical treatments can suffer post-traumatic symptoms. These procedures are often worse for children, especially if they occurred in an era when parents were routinely separated from their sick children. Suzanne describes how her experience of forced separation from her family at age five influenced choices she made as a mother:

> I never really thought about why I chose to give up a promising career to stay home with my three children. It was made easier since it was economically feasible for us. But later, as I thought about my own mostly happy childhood, I found I am still saddened by the one dark time I encountered.
>
> When I was five years old, I contracted polio and was separated from my family for almost a full year in two separate hospitals. We were allowed occasional family visits, but only every other Sunday for two hours. It was just not enough time to get rid of those fears of abandonment. I knew deep down in my heart that I would go home, but was still fearful, since I didn't have any idea when. It still haunts me today as I feel for that scared little girl.

Sometimes, the illness and death of a mother or father can change family dynamics and lead to some difficulties for the children. If your mother died during your childhood, you may have found it necessary to be the caregiver while you were still young. While this is understandable, it still could be influencing how you feel. For many years, we've known that children whose mother dies, especially when the child is younger than thirteen, are at increased risk of depression throughout their lives. Grief is certainly part of the reason, but there may also be something else going on. Researchers are now wondering if children's reactions could also be due to inadequate care prior to their mothers' deaths (Bifulco et al. 1992).

Long-term Effects of Past Abuse

While not everyone who experienced child maltreatment shows symptoms, the effects can continue well into adulthood. This section summarizes some of the effects you might have experienced or are experiencing now. Sometimes, parenting your own child will make memories of these past experiences very vivid. The long-term effects of past abuse can also affect your psychological and physical health, both of which can influence how you mother your own children.

Sometimes children show very functional coping behaviors in childhood (such as seeking the assistance of a supportive adult), and do not show symptoms of past abuse as adults. Other times, their coping abilities are less positive, and the symptoms adult survivors manifest are often logical extensions of dysfunctional coping mechanisms developed during childhood (Briere and Elliot 1994). While these dysfunctional behaviors may have helped you cope with ongoing abuse when you were a child, they often have a negative impact on adult functions. Researchers John Briere and Diana Elliot have divided the long-term effects of childhood maltreatment into six domains. This framework may help you understand those effects in your own life. I have added a seventh domain (physical health).

Post-Traumatic Stress Disorder (PTSD)

The diagnosis of post-traumatic stress disorder (PTSD) came about as a result of clinicians' work with Vietnam veterans. It has since been applied to many other types of traumatic events as well: many adult survivors of physical, sexual, or severe emotional abuse show symptoms of PTSD. To receive a formal diagnosis of PTSD, a person must have experienced a discernible traumatic event, such as past sexual abuse, and display the following symptoms:

1. Frequent reexperiencing of the event via nightmares or intrusive thoughts

2. Numbing, or lack of responsiveness to or avoidance of current events

3. Persistent symptoms of increased arousal, including jumpiness, sleep disturbance, or poor concentration

Briere and Elliot note that many abuse survivors have symptoms of PTSD even if they do not meet the full criteria for a formal diagnosis. For example, they estimate that 80 percent of sexual abuse survivors have some post-traumatic symptoms. These symptoms include hypervigilance, intrusive thoughts, and flashbacks.

Flashbacks can be triggered by a variety of stimuli, including current abuse by another adult, talking to someone else about your abusive experiences, or learning of the abusive experiences of others. They can also be triggered by tactile or sensory stimuli associated with the abuse, such as smells (e.g., the scent of a particular cologne), tastes, textures, or sounds.

For some adult survivors of child sexual abuse, birth experiences can trigger flashbacks. Possible triggers related to birth include physical pain, callous treatment by caregivers, perceived loss of control, or the perineal pressure of second-stage labor. As noted in one qualitative study, birth can suddenly revive memories of sexual abuse that make it seem as if it was happening right then (Rhoades and Hutchinson 1994).

Childhood abuse can also increase your vulnerability to stresses you may experience as an adult. In one study, Vietnam veterans who had been physically abused as children were found to be significantly more likely to develop post-traumatic stress disorder PTSD after combat than were veterans who had not been abused as children (Bremner et al. 1993). These findings were true even when the researchers compared veterans who had had the same amount of combat exposure.

What this means for you is that a previously abusive experience, of whatever type, may increase your risk for having a traumatic-stress reaction to something that happens to you in adulthood. Experiences that could trigger this reaction include being mugged or assaulted as an adult, having a frightening birth experience, or the serious illness of someone in your family (including you or your child).

Cognitive Distortions

If you experienced abuse in childhood, you may see the world as a dangerous place. Because you have been powerless in the past, you may be highly fearful and tend to overestimate danger and adversity in your current environment. In dealing with both real and perceived danger, you may feel there is nothing you can do. You may feel powerless to protect and provide for your children. Cognitive distortions can also influence what you think about your child. In one recent study, mothers who had been physically abused had significantly more negative thoughts about their babies than did the comparison mothers, who had not been physically abused (Gara 2000). These distortions can contribute to your emotional distress and increase your risk for depression.

Emotional Distress

Another category of symptoms is emotional distress, including depression, anxiety, and anger. Depression is the most commonly reported symptom of past abuse.

Adult survivors have a four-times-greater lifetime risk for a major depressive episode than adults who have not been abused or neglected (Johnson et al. 1999). Some of this vulnerability to depression has a physiological basis. Severe or chronic stressors may alter the way your brain handles stressful events, leaving you more vulnerable to depression when confronted with a current life stress (Weiss et al. 1999).

Adult survivors of abuse are also at risk to experience anxiety disorders, panic disorders, phobias, and obsessive-compulsive disorder (OCD). These anxiety-related symptoms are frequently associated with PTSD responses and cognitive distortions. Anxiety can be made worse by a negative birth experience, or by having a baby who is born premature, ill, or disabled. These birth-related experiences, or the ongoing illness of your children, may make you very fearful.

Anger, another symptom of emotional distress, includes chronic irritability, rage, and difficulties in expressing anger in a constructive way. Survivors may suppress their anger to such an extent that they feel they have no right to be angry with their partner, coworkers, friends, or children. These suppressed feelings may eventually explode.

Claire describes how her molestation as a child affected her ability to mother her son. In the immediate postpartum period and for the first year, she felt overwhelming sadness and grief. Later, she found herself feeling very angry. Her story begins with her follow-up visits to her midwife:

> Over the next days and weeks, I had several follow-up visits. Some were routine, but a few were because I just had a lot of trouble breastfeeding. Then too, I was glad of the contact with the midwives because I just couldn't stop crying. I felt bursting with pride at this incredible thing I'd done, and yet all I could feel when I looked at that perfect

little one was grief, grief, grief. I could not understand it. The emotions were so intense that I could not sort them out or make them calm down.

Eventually I wore out. I wouldn't say I felt peaceful. I just felt like a dry autumn leaf. Resigned. Powdery. Light-weight. Just waiting to blow away or disintegrate. And by turns I began to feel normal things too, like fatigue, humor, boredom, longing for grown-ups to talk to, long-ing to go to work again, longing for a baby-sitter. It is true that there was a sort of gap between how I'd envisioned myself mothering and how I was managing in reality. But I think this is normal. I felt normal.

Then there came that time when they start to have a will of their own, and they sometimes cry in anger, assert-ing themselves. And it terrified me. When he out-and-out cried like that I'd fill with adrenaline as though my life were in danger—as though his life were in danger. I was afraid I'd hit him or shake him to get him to stop it, so I'd find myself sitting outside on the front stoop while he wailed in the safety of his crib.

Other things start being obviously "not right" then too. I sometimes would cry uncontrollably and feel nause-ated. I'd spend whole days lying on my bed while he was at day care. I felt the gap between how I wanted to be with him and how I seemed to be as a mother widening. And then came some way, way stronger-than-usual reactions to things that were related to my memories of being molested: adrenaline rushes and strange sensations and panic and dread. I started to feel as though I were "losing it," or worse. Maybe I was becoming mentally ill, like my mother.

Impaired Sense of Self

Women who have experienced childhood abuse often have an impaired sense of self. You may use the reactions of others to gauge how you are feeling about a particular situation. Because of this, you may be gullible and easily manipulated by others. You may be unable to establish appropriate boundaries, even with your children, and are often the caretaker of others within your network of friends and family. An impaired sense of self can also increase your risk of revictimization, including rape or domestic abuse. Finally, you may have difficulty asking others for help, gathering a support network, or taking advantage of support that is available. This difficulty can have direct implications for your emotional well-being and your ability to mother.

Avoidance

Avoidance is another long-term effect of abuse—one that is at the heart of many of the more serious symptoms. Avoidance symptoms can occur because they help you cope by temporarily reducing emotional pain. One type of avoidance is dissociation. Dissociative symptoms often first appear during childhood, when they become a way to "escape" from abuse or pain. Adult survivors often describe how they were able to numb body parts at will, or how they would "watch" the abuse from outside their body. Some mothers can still use dissociation to cope with uncomfortable feelings of intense contact with their babies or children. Dissociation gets to be a problem for these mothers, however, when they have no control over when it happens.

Numbing of body parts and other types of dissociative reactions can also take place during birth. In a qualitative analysis of adult survivors during labor, Rhoades and Hutchinson (1994) describe how some of the women they studied would remove themselves mentally and emotionally from labor. These women appeared to have "easy" labors in that they did not cry out or indicate that they were experiencing a great deal of pain. However, the nurses and midwives who attended them were concerned because the mothers appeared to be "absent" from their bodies. These types of dissociative responses may also be present when a mother breastfeeds.

Amnesia for abuse-related events is another type of avoidance response. Not everyone experiences amnesia, but many do. Linda Williams, of Wellesley College, conducted a prospective study (1994) of adults who, when they were children, had been treated for sexual assault in an emergency room of a large urban hospital. When she recontacted these women twenty years later, she found that 38 percent of the women she interviewed—all of whom had confirmed and documented sexual abuse experiences—had experienced total or partial amnesia regarding their abuse experiences. If you have large blocks of your childhood that you cannot remember, you may have had a traumatic experience in your life. It is normal to remember back to ages three or four. When someone tells me that they cannot remember anything before the age of thirteen, for example, I find it is almost invariably a sign of some type of major childhood trauma. Gwen describes how memories of her abuse experience came flooding back once her child reached the same age she was when her abuse began:

> The first time I had issues with my abuse and raising my son was when he was five. This was the same age when I remembered my abuse beginning. I freaked out the entire year. I was afraid to give him a bath or touch him in any way. I would have thoughts about abusing him. At this time, I was in individual therapy, and there I learned that all this was okay as long as I did not act on it. I believe if I ever get to that point I will commit myself somewhere for help.

Not surprisingly, women who have had abuse experiences as children are more likely to abuse substances, engage in dangerous sexual liaisons, have eating disorders, and injure themselves—including multiple suicide attempts. All of these behaviors can endanger you and your children. If you are having trouble with any of these, it's important to seek professional mental health treatment immediately.

Interpersonal Problems

Adult survivors of past abuse may also experience difficulties in relationships with others, including partners, friends, members of their family of origin, and their children. Evvie Becker-Lausen and Sharon Mallon-Kraft (1997) describe two dysfunctional interpersonal styles that they characterize as "pandemic" outcomes of past abuse. Adult survivors may adopt an "avoidant" style, which involves low interdependency, self-disclosure, and warmth, and leaves the survivor with few interpersonal ties. Or they may adopt an "intrusive" style, which involves extremely high needs for closeness, excessive self-disclosure, and a tendency to be smotheringly warm, overly demanding, and controlling. If you're familiar with the concept of codependency, you may notice its similarity with the intrusive style. You'll also notice that the two styles are very similar to those of depressed mothers. Interestingly, both styles result in loneliness.

Past abuse influences adult relationships. In a sample of incest survivors, those not in stable or secure relationships as adults were more likely to be depressed (Alexander et al. 1998). Past abuse can influence your ability to trust others, make friends, and have relationships that are not exploitive. Adult survivors are often isolated and are less satisfied with their relationships than adults who were never abused. If you are an abuse survivor, you may find it difficult to find

---

WILL YOU ABUSE YOUR OWN KIDS?

A question I'm often asked is whether adult survivors are likely to abuse their own children. Adult survivors are at increased risk for abusing their children, but most do not.

Researchers have identified three protective factors that kept mothers from abusing their own children:

1. Emotional support from at least one nonabusive adult during childhood
2. Participation in therapy at some point
3. A stable, satisfying relationship as an adult

Mothers with one or more of these protective factors were more often able to break the cycle of abuse (Buist 1998; Egeland et al. 1988; Zuravin et al. 1996).

---

an adequate support network to help you cope with the stresses of parenting.

Physical Health Problems

The symptoms discussed so far have been related to emotional and mental health. Childhood abuse and trauma can have a fairly dramatic effect on physical health as well. Women who have experienced traumatic events go to the doctor more, report more health symptoms, and, in our study, had surgery twice as often as a comparison group who did not report past abuse (Kendall-Tackett et al. 2000). We also found that abuse survivors were more vulnerable to stress-related illnesses, such as diabetes. Fatigue and weakness were also common (Kendall-Tackett and Marshall 1999).

Chronic pain was one of the most commonly reported symptoms. The flood of stress hormones after a traumatic event sensitizes the body, and actually appears to lower the pain threshold, making sensations more painful. Pain syndromes related to past physical or sexual abuse are irritable bowel syndrome, chronic pelvic pain, frequent headaches, and fibromyalgia (Kendall-Tackett 2000).

What You Can Do

Past abuse can influence every area of your life, including how you mother your children. But there is much you can do to heal. Your past does not have to rule your future.

DIFFERENCES IN RESPONSE TO PAST ABUSE

Some people are deeply affected by past abuse, whereas others seem to show no symptoms at all. Your reaction could be anywhere along this spectrum. Not everyone who has experienced abuse will be traumatized. Researchers have identified several factors related to more severe reactions.

In general, abuse will be more harmful if the abuser was someone you knew and trusted. Your emotional attachment to the perpetrator and sense of betrayal can be more important predictors of harm than whether they are related to you. Another important factor is the severity of the abusive acts. For sexual abuse, severity is defined by whether the abuse experiences included penetration (oral, vaginal or anal). For physical abuse, severity is described in terms of damage and degree of injury: the more severe the abuse, the worse the injuries. For neglect, severity is described in terms of the degree of deprivation.

Abuse that occurs often and lasts for years will typically be more harmful than abuse that happens only sporadically and over less time. The exception is the one-time violent assault (Kendall-Tackett et al. 1993). Not surprisingly, use of force has been shown to increase the severity of reaction to sexual abuse. While all sexual abuse is, by definition, nonconsensual, sometimes the abuser will use trickery or mental coercion rather than force to gain compliance. In other situations, the abuser will hit, assault, or physically restrain his victim. Victims who experience this type of abuse are more likely to have symptoms, as are victims who have experienced multiple types of abuse.

Should You Just "Get Over It"?

For many years, the prevailing wisdom encouraged trauma survivors to "just forget about it." This advice still exists today, in the form of the flippantly delivered admonition to "get over it." But is that advice effective? Holocaust survivors are often used as examples of people who experienced horrifying events and yet put their pasts behind them. At first, they seemed to function well. However, as these same survivors hit the milestones of middle and old age, we find that their experiences start to haunt them. In a fascinating paper, researchers noted that as Holocaust survivors in their study aged, they had increasingly difficult experiences of their children leaving home and their own retirement and illness. The survivors had worse experiences of cancer. They had more pain. Hospitalizations were more traumatic. They experienced even political events, such as bombing during the Gulf War, more keenly than those who had not gone through the Holocaust (Solomon and Ginzburg 1999). The researchers noted that as these people aged, their level of busyness decreased, allowing traumatic memories to surface again.

In my community, I've been struck by the number of perimenopausal women who have experienced difficulties from past traumatic events. Of course, their medical care providers have attributed this to hormones. And there may in fact be a physiologic basis for some of these symptoms. But it is also possible that as child care needs were becoming less intense these women's memories of traumatic events came back in force. In sum, the "get over it" strategy appears to work only temporarily, which leads me to my next suggestion.

Process Your Experience

In order to heal, you must find a way to process your traumatic experience. Professional therapy is one good way to do so. Remember that participating in therapy is one factor that prevents people from abusing their own children. Therapy can be either individual (just you and the therapist) or in groups (a small group of people with similar issues, under a therapist's guidance). Be sure to seek out someone who has experience treating past abuse. State psychological associations can often give referrals. It's also important to find someone you like and have rapport with. Sharing your secret with someone can be remarkably healing in and of itself.

One area to specifically address in therapy is the presence of cognitive distortions. During your abuse experience, you may have internalized messages about being stupid, lazy, or dirty, and these thoughts could be influencing you today. Much of the harm that comes from past abusive experiences is directly related to what you tell yourself about it.

Another way to process traumatic events is through writing. The research of James Pennebaker demonstrates the powerful healing effects of expressing emotions in writing. Many of the men and women in his studies went through experiences similar to yours. Once they wrote about their experiences for a certain amount of time, they were able to put their traumatic pasts behind them. This resulted in measurable improvements in their psychological and physical health. If you want to give journaling a try, I'd encourage you to get Pennebaker's book, *Opening Up* (1997), since it has many specific suggestions to help you get the most out of this activity.

Get Support

The process of recovery from traumatic events can take a long time. It's helpful if you have people in your life who understand that, and will give you the space to heal. Having the support of others who have gone through similar experiences can also be important.

Support is especially important if you are irritable, withdrawn, or having difficulties controlling your anger. All of these can be symptoms of depression, a common occurrence among adult survivors. If you feel like lashing out at your child, or are feeling detached, you need to find someone to help you through these times. Be realistic about how much responsibility you take on. You may feel resentful when your children don't appreciate all the hard work that you are doing on their behalf, or how much better their childhood is than yours. When you are in danger of blowing your top, call someone. Most cities have chapters of Parents Anonymous or other "warmlines." These numbers are in the front of your phone book; use them when you need them.

You might also consider seeking out one or more mothering mentors. Many times, adult survivors have no idea how to parent since their own upbringing was so difficult. We all tend to parent as we were parented. If you want to break the cycle of abuse, find someone who can help. To find a mentor, seek out women who seem to have good relationships with their children and have a positive view of mothering. Ask for their advice. If they offer their opinion in a way that makes you feel respected, continue to seek them out.

Special Considerations for the Breastfeeding Mother

Adult survivors of physical and sexual abuse face a whole range of additional challenges when they breastfeed. The intense physical contact of breastfeeding may be very uncomfortable for you. You might find breastfeeding painful because your abuse experience lowered your pain threshold. The act of breastfeeding may also trigger flashbacks.

Some mothers I've spoken with breastfeed because they think it's best for the baby, but they hate it the whole time. Other mothers find that the breast pump makes them very uncomfortable. I some-times meet mothers who feel that they must do whatever their chil-dren want with regard to breastfeeding, even if it makes them cringe.

Several years ago, I gave one of my first talks on breastfeeding and the sexual abuse survivor. The next day a young woman approached me who had breastfed three children, two of whom were still nursing. She asked me if she would ever like it. I truthfully didn't know how to answer. Since that time, many other mothers have told me that while it was never great, breastfeeding became more tolerable over time.

If you are an abuse survivor who is struggling with breastfeed-ing, I have some specific suggestions. First, try to figure out what sit-uations make you feel uncomfortable. Is it nighttime feeding? Is it your baby touching other parts of your body while nursing? Is it the latch-on? Second, try to make these problem areas better. If skin-to-skin contact is bothering you, can you put a towel between you and the baby? Can you avoid the feedings (perhaps nighttime feedings) that make you uncomfortable? Would you be more com-fortable if you pumped and fed your baby with a bottle? Can you hold your baby's hand while nursing to keep him from touching other parts of your body? Can you distract yourself while nursing with TV or a book? (Many mothers have told me that this works well for them.) Experiment and find out what helps.

And third, remember that some breastfeeding is better than none—even if you must pump milk and use a bottle, or you are only nursing once a day. If you find yourself feeling rage while nursing, it's probably better for you and your baby if you stop. Mothering is not about martyrdom. If breastfeeding is something you loathe, don't do it. Remember too that you don't owe other people an explanation for the choices you make. It's none of their business (tell them I said so).

Set Some Boundaries

As a child, you may have had others violate your boundaries over and over. Now that you are an adult, you may have difficulties saying no to others. This may happen with your children, your part-ner, or other adults. Our culture pressures all mothers to do too much. But abuse survivors often feel a double portion of pressure, since they are unable to place reasonable limits on how much time and energy they give to others. Learning to set such boundaries can have a major impact on the quality of your life. See chapter 3 and

Henry Cloud and John Townsend's book *Boundaries* (1992) for some more specific suggestions.

Visualize Your Capacity for Wellness

I started studying family violence in 1983. At that time, I was an intern at one of the first treatment programs in the country for incest survivors. Many of the men and women there were very symptomatic, having endured the most extreme forms of abuse. During a training session, one of the senior clinicians said something that I never forgot. She said that we must always see the capacity for wellness in our clients. We must see this, and communicate it to them. The therapist who said this had seen people with very severe manifestations of past abuse, and yet she was able to hold out this hope.

Your experience of childhood abuse has most likely had an impact on you. But what started as a difficulty can be turned into a strength. Adult survivors have reported that eventually, good came from their experiences (McMillen et al. 1995). They described how their abusive pasts made them more sensitive to the needs of others. Many felt compelled to help others who had suffered similar experiences. You can indeed become strong in the broken places.

Conclusion

Reactions to past abuse vary from person to person. The responses of some survivors are relatively mild, while others experience severe reactions. Even when the abusive experience produced severe trauma, however, there is hope for healing. Your life can be good.

For Further Reading

There are many good books and other resources available to help you overcome the negative effects of past abuse. You are not alone.

Resources for Processing Your Traumatic Experience

This is a small sampling of materials that are available. Most books on the market are for survivors of sexual abuse, but there are also books on other types of maltreatment and family dysfunction.

Bowden, J. D., H. L. Gravitz, and S. W. Cruse. 1987. *Recovery: A Guide for Adult Children of Alcoholics.* New York: Fireside.

Copeland, M. E., and M. Harris. 2000. *Healing the Trauma of Abuse: A Women's Workbook.* Oakland, Calif.: New Harbinger.

Courtois, C. A. 1996. *Healing the Incest Wound: Adult Survivors in Therapy.* New York: W. W. Norton.

Matsakis, A. 1996. *I Can't Get Over It: A Handbook for Trauma Survivors.* Oakland, Calif.: New Harbinger.

———. 1998. *Trust After Trauma: A Guide to Relationships for Survivors and Those Who Love Them.* Oakland, Calif.: New Harbinger.

Pennebaker, J. W. 1997. *Opening Up: The Healing Power of Expressing Emotions.* New York: Guilford Press.

Salter, A. C. 1995. *Transforming Trauma: A Guide to Understanding and Treating Adult Survivors of Child Sexual Abuse.* Newbury Park, Calif.: Sage Publications.

Seixas, J. S., and G. Yoncha. 1986. *Children of Alcoholics: A Survivor's Manual.* New York: HarperTrade.

Sperlich, M. *Survivor Moms Speak Out.* Mickey Sperlich is a midwife in Michigan who has been compiling a book for mothers who are abuse survivors. Her book was still in progress as this one went to press, but she said readers could contact her for ordering information. New Moon Midwifery, newmoonmid@aol.com

Information and Support for Past Abuse

Adult Survivors of Child Abuse: www.ascasupport.org
Healing Journey Chat Rooms for Adult Survivors of Trauma and Abuse: www.healing-journey.net
Rape, Abuse and Incest National Network: www.rainn.org

Adult Children of Alcoholics

Adult Children of Alcoholics World Service Organization: www.adultchildren.org
Children of Alcoholics Foundation: www.coaf.org
National Association for Children of Alcoholics: www.nacoa.net

Domestic Violence

National Organization for Victim Assistance: www.try-nova.org
Safe Horizon: www.safehorizon.org

Books about Psychological Trauma in General

These are great books to read if you want a broader understanding of psychological trauma in general. You may be surprised (and reassured) to discover that many of the emotions you are experiencing are predictable and normal for people who have experienced negative or stressful life events.

Briere, J. N. 1992. *Child Abuse Trauma: Theory and Treatment of the Lasting Effects*. Newbury Park, Calif.: Sage Publications.

Figley, C. 1985. *Trauma and Its Wake: The Study and Treatment of Post-Traumatic Stress Disorder*. New York: Bruner/Mazel.

Figley, C. 1986. *Trauma and Its Wake: Vol II. Traumatic Stress, Theory, Research and Intervention*. New York: Bruner/Mazel.

Herman, J. L. 1992. *Trauma and Recovery*. New York: Basic Books.

CHAPTER 9

CHALLENGING CHILD I
MOTHERING A CHILD WITH BEHAVIORAL ISSUES

A couple of years ago, I was waiting for my son at a soccer camp. Soon, another mom joined me. As we chatted, she proceeded to tell me about her "hyper" son. On several occasions, she apologized in advance for her child's behavior, anticipating that he would soon be acting up. Although we had just met, she shared with me how mothering her challenging child had undermined her confidence, isolated her from other parents, strained her marriage, and kept her from having more children. And she is not alone.

Children with behavioral issues can push parents to their limits. A recent article published in the journal *Child Abuse & Neglect* demonstrates the seriousness of problems that parents can face. In Sullivan and Knutson's study (2000) of over 50,000 children in the Midwest, they found that children with behavioral disorders were *seven times* more likely to be maltreated (neglected and physically and emotionally abused) than were children without behavioral difficulties. Much of this abuse occurred in their own homes, and 67 percent of the abusers were mothers.

In this chapter, I describe two types of behavioral difficulties: the spirited temperament, and attention deficit hyperactivity disorder (ADHD). While temperament and attentional difficulties are two distinct entities, they sometimes overlap, and share many similarities in terms of how they make mothers feel. I focus on behavior because it is the most salient, and challenging, aspect of mothering these children.

The Spirited Temperament

From the start, babies come to us with their own personalities or temperaments, which range from easy to difficult. It is the "difficult" child who is the subject of this section. You may have noticed that I did not use "difficult" in the title for this section. Mary Kurcinka, author of *Raising Your Spirited Child* (1991), points out that the word "difficult" emphasizes the negative aspects of this personality type without describing any of the positives. She prefers the term "spirited" because it honestly captures the challenges you face, while also describing the strengths of these children. It is a term that can give both you and your child hope.

What Is a Spirited Child?

Children's temperaments include several dimensions: how much they cry, how well they adapt to new situations, how irritable they are, how active they are, and so on. Kurcinka (1991) lists nine dimensions that describe the spirited temperament; your child's temperament might exhibit one or more (or even all) of these dimensions:

1. **Intense.** Spirited children are intense. They often react negatively and tend to cry frequently, and when they do, it is loud. Positive emotions are powerful (and loud) too.

2. **Persistent.** Spirited children are also persistent. Once they "lock in" to an activity, they are reluctant to give it up.

3. **Sensitive.** These children are highly sensitive to sounds, smells, and the feel of their clothing. They become easily overwhelmed by crowds or lots of sensations at once. When their senses are overloaded, they have a tendency to overreact and have tantrums, both at home and in public places.

4. **Perceptive.** Spirited children notice everything, and must often stop to observe whatever catches their attention. They may be on their way to do one thing when they get distracted by something else.

5. **Not easily adaptable.** Spirited children can be slow to accept new experiences. They do not enjoy surprises, and often have difficulty transitioning from one activity to another.

6. **Irregular.** These children tend not to engage in regular routines. They are almost impossible to get on any kind of

schedule. Many of them are also almost super-human in their lack of need for sleep. Of course, this trait alone contributes to many of the bad feelings that mothers of these children experience.

7. **Energetic.** Children with spirited temperaments are also often on the high end of the energy scale. Even if they are not running around, they are busy taking things apart, exploring, or making things.

8. **Tend to have a negative first reaction.** Spirited children will often receive new situations or activities negatively. Their first reaction is often "no."

9. **Tend to have gloomy mood.** Spirited children can be very serious or even gloomy. They can also be pessimistic, and are likely to focus on the negative aspects or flaws of a situation.

It's helpful to think of these dimensions as continua. Even among children with spirited temperaments, there is variation. Your child may have a personality that is mildly spirited, or your child may be on the other end—what some have called "explosive."

Children with spirited temperaments can push mothers to their limits, even while they are still babies. Anthropologist Sheila Kitzinger studied 1,400 women in Australia and England. She compared mothers of babies who cried the most (more than six hours per day) to babies who cried the least (less than two hours per day). Among the mothers whose babies cried the most, she found that 80 percent were depressed, 57 percent described "desperate need to escape," 50 percent admitted that they were "itching to smack the baby," and 33 percent made negative comments about their partners. Common themes these mothers shared were of feeling trapped, or guilty, useless, exhausted, inadequate, and bewildered (Kitzinger 1990). In introducing these findings, Kitzinger made an interesting observation. She said that prior to working on this study, she couldn't understand how anyone could hit a baby. After the study, she was *amazed* that these women managed so much self-control.

As infants, spirited children need to be held a great deal of the time. They often will not separate from you. If you leave them with a sitter, they may cry the whole time you are gone. These needs can leave you feeling drained. They also open you up to criticism from others who assume that you *made* your child this way.

As your spirited child matures, she may not cry so much. But she will continue to exhibit behavior that exasperates you. Your feelings of frustration often will continue even with older children, as Lynn describes:

> I have a three-and-a-half-year-old spirited child. He is highly intelligent and very articulate. But he has a very two-sided disposition. He can be the most thoughtful, generous, loving, helping child. He can also be your worst nightmare. He bites other children to get his way. He must always win every confrontation. When he is in his bad mood, he will do anything to be difficult. He truly does not care about what the cost will be, and once he is in this mode, I can't get him out of it. My husband has a particularly difficult time with him when he is this way.

SHOULD YOU LET YOUR BABY "CRY IT OUT"?

Parents of spirited children are often advised to let their babies cry. If you respond to your child's cries, the thinking goes, you are "reinforcing" it. If you have already tried this advice, you most likely know that it doesn't work well for children with spirited temperaments. As Robert Wright describes in an article on parent-child cosleeping (1997), his first child could cry for two hours straight "without reloading." Spirited children can become overwhelmed by their own strong emotions. For them, crying can last for hours rather than minutes. It's not unusual for spirited children to become so upset while they cry that they throw up.

Does responding to crying "reinforce" it? Technically "reinforcement" refers to increasing the likelihood that the behavior will occur. So the idea is that if you respond to crying, the baby will be more likely to cry in the future. Interestingly, researchers have found the opposite to be true (Cassidy and Shaver 1999). For example, when mothers in one study consistently responded to and tried to comfort their crying babies at three months (Crockenberg and McCluskey 1986), the babies (including those with difficult temperaments) cried less during separation at twelve months and were more securely attached.

Factors That Can Influence How You Feel

Spirited children are not all equal. Each child is a unique person, in a unique family, with unique circumstances. But some types of situations are more difficult than others, making things more challenging for you.

Sleep Deprivation

A spirited temperament is often obvious from birth. These children can be poor sleepers and don't seem to require as much sleep as other children their age. If you have a baby or child who wakes several times during the night, this alone can wreak havoc on your emotional state. As I frequently tell mothers, prisoners of war are deprived of sleep as a means of *torture*. Therefore, you shouldn't be surprised when you fare poorly on limited sleep. (See chapter 7 for some specific suggestions to help you cope.)

Excessive Disruptiveness

Your child's behavior is going to be more difficult for you if it includes tantrums, outbursts, screaming, running around, and aggression toward children or adults. These disruptive behaviors can draw unwanted attention to you and your child. Your child's disruptiveness can also be isolating for you.

Loss of Self-esteem and Confidence in Parenting

What you think about your child's behaviors also makes a difference. Much of the anguish of mothering a child with a spirited temperament comes from inside your own mind. If you blame yourself for this behavior, your experience of it will be worse than if you attribute it to your child's personality. Mothers with other, nonspirited children are more likely to recognize the importance of temperament than are mothers with only one, spirited child. Similarly, mothers with a more laid-back style of mothering are going to be more comfortable than mothers who want to be on top of everything in their lives.

Lack of Support

Support makes a difference here too. Mothers who have other people in their lives who encourage them and offer to help fare better physically and emotionally than mothers who have no one or, worse, lots of criticism.

In the next section, I describe the child with ADHD. There is a substantial amount of overlap between a spirited temperament and ADHD, and some children have characteristics of both. But these are separate entities.

Attention-Deficit/Hyperactivity Disorder (ADHD)

You can spot them quickly: the kids who just can't sit still or pay attention. Parents and teachers say that they are "hyper." Children with attention-deficit/hyperactivity disorder (ADHD) often do draw attention to themselves by acting up and getting in trouble, both at school and at home.

ADHD actually refers to several different chronic disorders, and is estimated to occur in approximately 3 to 5 percent of school-age children. It is two to three times more likely to occur in boys (National Institute of Mental Health 2000a). However, when "hyper-activity" is dropped from the list of symptoms, the number of boys and girls is near equal. The number of diagnoses of ADHD is on the rise, as is its impact on the healthcare system. In 1990, a survey of 2,400 practicing physicians indicated that there were 2 million patient visits associated with ADHD. By 1994, this number had reached 4.7 million (Sears and Thompson 1998).

In the introduction to *The A.D.D. Book*, pediatrician William Sears describes three types of children he sees in his practice that have a diagnosis of attention-deficit disorder (ADD). The first are children with a true biological anomaly that causes them to think, act, and learn differently. For these children, he recommends a three-pronged management approach that includes medication, behavioral strategies, and learning strategies. The second type of child has a "situational" type of ADD. These children's symptoms are manifest only in some settings (such as a classroom), and generally reflect a mismatch between the situation and the child's needs. Finally, there are children who are bright, energetic, and creative who act, and learn differently but do not have a disability. However, these children are often inconvenient for teachers with large classes and schools that value sameness. According to Sears, these children do not deserve a label, but need a learning environment that meets their needs. Along these lines, some more alternative-oriented physicians such as Andrew Weil wonder whether we are too quick to attach a label of ADHD to any child, usually a boy, who is active (Weil 2000). Is it really ADHD or just normal development?

Symptoms of ADHD

There are four core symptoms of ADHD. Your child may have any or all of these. The first is **inattention**. An inattentive child has difficulty concentrating and gets bored easily. Such children often have difficulty completing assignments and routine tasks because their attention wanders or they are easily distracted.

The second symptom is **selective attention**. Children with ADHD can become hyperfocused on one thing, ignoring everything else. Selective attention explains why children who have difficulty completing assignments can play video games for hours. As I'll describe later, this hyperfocus can also be a strength. But it can be a problem for your child if it is not properly channeled.

The next symptom is **hyperactivity**. Not all children with an attentional disorder have this symptom. Hyperactive children are always in motion. Even when these children are sitting, they are tapping their feet or a pencil. They wiggle and roam around the room, and have a tendency to talk incessantly. It can be one of the more difficult symptoms for you and others to cope with. Attentional difficulties without this symptom (ADD rather than ADHD) are often not diagnosed because the children are not disruptive in class. Some of their lack of attention might be misinterpreted as "laziness" or lack of motivation.

The final core symptom is **impulsivity**. Children with this symptom seem unable to control their behavior, and often do not think before they act. They may hit, blurt out inappropriate information, have a hard time waiting for their turn in games, and grab toys from other children. They also have a tendency to lose or break things, and can be accident-prone (National Institute of Mental Health 2000b). These characteristics often make children appear less mature than their peers, and can make them targets for bullies at school (Sears and Thompson 1998).

Some other traits that have been observed in children with ADHD are similar to traits described earlier regarding temperament. The first is intensity. These children are often described as being "too emotional" by teachers and others. Related to this are tendencies to overreact, and to be unaffected by past consequences or future rewards. These children often have poor handwriting. They need frequent rewards and are more likely to find many things "boring" (Sears and Thompson 1998).

Factors That Influence How You Feel

Life with a child with ADHD can present many challenges similar to those of parenting a spirited child. Here are some of the factors that can influence how you feel.

Disruptive Behavior

The more disruptive the behavior of a child with ADHD, the more challenging mothering will be for you. You may be embarrassed to take your child anywhere since you don't know how he'll act. Your child may grab toys from others and act up at relatives' homes. You may have difficulty getting your child through the school system, and find yourself frequently meeting with school personnel. It may be impossible for you to just go somewhere without making extensive plans.

Strenuousness of the Treatment Regimen

Another factor influencing how you feel is the difficulty of your child's ADHD treatment regimen. You may find that a multipronged approach works best, and this routine may include dietary modifications, medications, and behavior management. For example, your child might be sensitive to artificial colors, flavors, or sugar. Unfortunately, all of these things are in foods children love. It can be a challenge to identify dietary sensitivities and monitor these foods.

If your child is on medication, it may take several attempts to find the right medication or dose that works for your child. Older children may skip medications or start refusing them. Multiple daily dosings are going to be more complex than a single dose. You may also have to arrange for medication to be given at school.

Finally, behavioral management also requires some intense planning. You may have to anticipate situations that set your child off, design rewards for good behavior, and help your child navigate some problem times.

Lack of Support

It will probably come as no surprise to you that support is important for mothers of children with ADHD. Mothers without support have a much harder time than mothers with support. You might blame yourself for your child's behaviors, and others may assume it's your fault too. You need people in your life who can counter some of this negative input and offer you some concrete support and assistance.

Living with ADHD: One Mother's Story

Below is an excerpt from Brandi Valentine's story (2000) of life with a son with ADHD. You'll notice some of the themes described earlier in this chapter. Her son's behaviors strained her relationships with her family of origin and her partner, who eventually left. Her son also had difficulties with other children and at school.

> By the time James was three, he had a "reputation." He had problems playing with other children. Older children, including his cousins and older sister, refused to play with him, so he spent much of his time playing alone. On the occasions he did play with other children, they were always younger than he was.
>
> James was often in trouble with the neighbors, and the fighting with his sister was nonstop. My father was the least understanding of all the family members, telling everyone that James was going to be the first family member ever to go to prison. He felt that if I just beat the kid, he'd straighten up. It got to be so that every visit to my parents deteriorated into a fight over my parenting skills and my lack of willingness to beat the child. My father hit James whenever James didn't conform to my father's wishes. Soon, the visits stopped. Things at home were not much better. The constant bickering between James and his sister was intense. James' father criticized me for my lack of ability to control the child and belittled me for my "poor parenting skills."
>
> When James was four, I was able to get him into a preschool class offered by the public school system. His behavior problems became more apparent and new behaviors arose as he was put into a classroom setting. The diagnosis from his preschool teachers: "Your child is psychotic." So I went to my pediatrician. He told me James was fine, but if I so desired he could put me on a waiting list for therapy. I was then sent home.
>
> At the age of five, James went to kindergarten. His ADD/ADHD behaviors became more pronounced. He could not perform such simple functions as cutting, drawing, or writing. He couldn't sit in his seat. He often spent his four hours a day in class either lying on the floor under the table, or wandering aimlessly through the classroom

touching everything. He was unable to stay on task no matter what he chose to do. The teacher, overwhelmed with thirty children, had no time for James, and as long as he didn't bother other students, he was allowed to wander through the class doing as he pleased. Due to the lack of funding in the school districts here, there was no aide for James' class, so I took on the role in order to help my son. It broke my heart to watch as he never got called upon to act out the little stories they learned. His papers were never placed on the wall, he was never invited to play with the other children, he was never chosen to take the attendance sheets to the office, and he was often left out of field trips because of his behavior. I now had something else to worry about—his self-esteem.

As Brandi's story indicates, ADHD can influence children's ability to make friends and do well in school. Such children's impulsiveness may lead to aggression with other children and may make them vulnerable to bullies. Other children may figure out how to make your child overreact, and he may end up in the principal's office—again! Your child may start to feel like a "bad kid." Not surprisingly, children with ADHD often have low self-esteem and are at higher risk for depression. If ADHD is unrecognized and untreated, children can have academic difficulties, increasing their risk of problems later in life, including problems with the law (Sears and Thompson 1998).

Some Common Feelings

If your child has a spirited temperament or attentional disorder, you are probably working a lot harder than other mothers. Even day-to-day tasks are more challenging. Simply getting dressed for the day may turn into a battle of wills, as your child insists on wearing shorts in 38–degree weather. If you forget to give your child adequate preparation for an upcoming change, you might find that he is "off" for the whole day. Even cutting a sandwich into squares instead of triangles can cause a meltdown.

Mothers of children with behavioral concerns receive lots of unsolicited child-rearing advice. This can make you feel resentful, misunderstood, or inadequate as a mother. The responsibilities of caring for a child with behavioral concerns can be overwhelming, as Ellen describes: "At one of our recent visits to our son's clinical psychologist, I was informed that if I were in a paid profession, I could probably to sue for 'burnout.'"

Depression

Mothers of children with behavioral concerns are also at higher risk for depression, and this risk starts in the child's infancy. One study found a direct link between a "difficult" temperament in babies and depression in mothers (Cutrona and Troutman 1986). These researchers also found that caring for a baby with a spirited temperament gradually eroded mothers' feelings of self-efficacy, making them feel incompetent. Another study found that depressed mothers tended to blame themselves for their infants' behaviors. This was despite the fact that the infants were *in reality* more "difficult" as determined by independent raters (Whiffen and Gotlib 1989).

Similarly, having a child with an attentional disorder can increase your vulnerability to depression (McCormick 1995). You may blame yourself for your child's difficulties and feel like you did something wrong. Even if you don't feel this way, others may openly speculate about what you did to bring about this condition in your child. Other families may not want you and your child around.

Without help and support, you might find yourself withdrawing from your baby or child, and describing him in mostly negative terms. Unfortunately, if this cycle is not interrupted, you might find yourself unhappy with your child most of the time and sometimes resorting to harsh forms of punishment, which ties in with the next reaction I describe: anger.

Anger

Another common reaction to dealing with a spirited or attention-disordered child is anger, and this may also start early in your relationship. Children who have behavioral problems can embarrass parents in public with tantrums or outbursts. They may be asked to leave play groups, day care, or preschool. They may bite or hit other children. Other parents can also get quite angry with your child. You may resent how much your child seems to need to be with you, and long for a break. Even during infancy, when these children don't sleep well, sleep deprivation may lead you to overreact to some of your child's behaviors. You might think about hitting your child, as Barbara describes:

When the baby started throwing up, I felt terrible. I wouldn't go anyplace with her because I didn't want people to see her screaming. I wanted to be the perfect mother. My mother-in-law said, "You've got to relax. She's picking up on your cues."

The baby had a difficult temperament. Even now, she's very stubborn and strong-willed. The control issue is big for me. I'm a perfectionist and always have been. I don't want the baby to experiment with food, even though I know it's normal.

I wanted this baby so bad. When she came, I hated her. I thought of throwing her out the window. I just wanted her to die. I spanked her when she was three or four weeks old, and I'm still dealing with the guilt of it. I'd yell at her, right in her face, "I hate you. I wish you would die."

As I mentioned earlier, children with behavioral difficulties are the most likely to be abused and neglected. It is important that you realize that many other parents experience anger at their children. But it is equally important that you get support and find safe ways to vent your anger so that it is not directed toward your child.

Guilt

Guilt is another common feeling among mothers of children with behavioral issues. Mothers tend to take a lot of responsibility for their children's behaviors. This may be especially true if the child with the behavioral issues is your first or only child. Mothers whose other children don't have behavioral concerns are often reassured that these behaviors are not their fault.

You may also feel guilty because you harbor some unpleasant feelings toward or even dislike your child. Sometimes, you might lose control and hit your child. When others talk to you about their warm feelings toward their children, you may begin to wonder what is wrong with you.

Isolation

Isolation is also common among parents of children with behavioral issues. Parents may find that they are socially shunned. Family outings may need to be limited because your child is easily overwhelmed by too many people in the room, too much noise, or too much visual distraction. You might also be embarrassed to go any-where with your child because you don't know how she will act. People will often let you know that you need to "do something," but will leave you to cope alone.

Your Other Relationships

Having a child with behavioral issues can influence your relation-ships. Your partner may imply, or actually say, that you need to do a better job controlling "your" child. You may find that all your time together as a couple is dominated by taking care of your child, with no time left to nurture your relationship with each other. The cumu-lative effect of months of sleep deprivation may make both of you overreact to real or imagined offenses. The stress on your marriage or relationship is real; divorce is twice as common in families with a child with ADHD as it is in families with no ADHD (Sears and Thompson 1998).

Caring for your child may severely limit other things you need to do. For example, if you are at home with your child, you may find it is difficult to even take a shower, let alone clean the house or pre-pare dinner. This can lead to many misunderstandings between you and your partner. Your partner may return home and wonder what you did all day. Mary, whose son has a temperament on the extreme end of spirited, described how in her family all other activities are on hold indefinitely. Her house is often in disarray, and one time was so "thrashed" that the cleaning service she had hired had to call the office for help. The whole situation may feel so overwhelming that you seek employment outside the home just so you can escape. Of course, you may find you have difficulties trying to find someone who will care for your child while you work.

Raising a child with a spirited temperament or ADHD can leave you feeling overwhelmed and drained. Right now, it's all you can do to cope day to day. It's impossible to even consider that there might be an upside. But there are parents who have raised children just like yours, and have lived to tell the tale.

Is There an Upside?

In the newest edition of the classic book *Parenting the Fussy Baby and the High-Need Child* (1996), William and Martha Sears open by describing their seventeen-year-old-daughter. She was their fussy baby, and the inspiration for their book. Now she is a bright, sensi-

tive, talented young woman. Spirited children often are very perceptive, insightful, and sensitive. They see and experience things more
deeply than do their more easygoing counterparts. The very characteristics that stress their parents actually turn into strengths.

Children with ADHD are also often very bright. Their ability to
hyperfocus can actually be an advantage in certain situations, such as
in sports. For example, it is a rare child who can concentrate so completely that she is not distracted by outside sights and sounds. The
ability to hyperfocus actually gives such a child a competitive edge.

High energy is another trait that can be trying for teachers and
parents. But these children can become highly productive adults.
Sears describes his own experiences as a child and an adult with
ADD. Even during medical school, his professors were concerned
about his high energy level. But he points out that he has written
twenty-three books and fathered eight children!

Finally, children with ADHD are also often very creative
because they are used to thinking about things differently. They can
think fast and are good at focusing on the "big picture." They can
also be very tenacious and persistent. While they may have difficulty
in school, they may excel at activities that require hands-on learning
and creativity.

What You Can Do

Fortunately, there are a number of positive steps you can take to live
more peacefully with your child. It is important that you take some
positive action. Without it, the issues these children face become
worse over time. Sears and Thompson (1998) note that ADHD that is
not recognized and managed can become a disability. If it is "understood, accepted, valued, and shaped" it can be an advantage for your
child and the people around him. A similar comment could be made
about children with spirited temperaments.

Become the Expert on Your Child

If you haven't already done so, learn everything you can about
your child's condition. This may mean reading parenting books,
searching the Internet, or joining a support group. Also, learn from
watching your child. When there is an "episode," try to figure out
what set things off after everything is calm again. You might find it
helpful to keep a log. Look for patterns, and try to figure out what
the triggers are for your child. Sears recommends that parents do this

because no one else will. Even if other people in your child's life care about him and want him to succeed, chances are they don't have the same investment that you have. Learn so that you can become your child's advocate.

Design Situations Where Your Child Can Win

Once you know what sets your child off, you can start to design situations that bring out the best in your child, instead of the worst. For example, you might limit your child's exposure to situations where there are lots of people he doesn't know, or where there is too much noise. You might start scheduling events, such as appointments or family outings, so that they occur during the time of day that is best for your child. Similarly, you might allow some acclimation time, or time between activities, so that you don't surprise your child with a sudden shift.

Sometimes, parents resent having to make all these accommodations for their children with behavioral challenges. Why must you go to all this extra effort on behalf of only one of your children? Others may have told you that your accommodations are silly, or will spoil your child. In considering whether these accommodations are a good idea, you might ponder what the alternative would be. You could try to force your child to behave, increase the amount and severity of punishment, or get into power struggles over everything. Chances are you have already tried this and found that it not only didn't work, but dramatically increased the degree of unpleasantness in your home.

Anticipating your child's trouble spots and doing some prevention does not mean that you will never have another unpleasant day. But you may find that the number decreases to a much more manageable level.

Avoid Power Struggles

A similar strategy has to do with avoiding battles over day-to-day activities by anticipating potential conflicts and having clear rules to deal with them. For example, you allow your child to select today's wardrobe, but you have only acceptable choices available. (If it is winter, store the shorts and tank tops elsewhere.) When asking what your child would like for breakfast, again offer only acceptable choices. You might offer "cold cereal or oatmeal." This avoids struggles that might arise when your child selects "candy" for breakfast because she was asked an open-ended question.

Make Correct Attributions for Your Child's Behavior

Many of the problems you encounter as a mother of a child with behavioral issues are due to what our culture has to say about children. Ours is a culture that values children's independence from a very early age. From birth, children sleep in their own beds and are encouraged to be as separate from you as possible. Any baby or child who protests this forced separation is said to be "manipulating" you.

However, children with spirited temperaments often have a very high need to be with you. They may not separate easily, and may cry until they make themselves sick. Parents put themselves and their children through these separations because it is thought to be in their children's best interests. Much of this cultural mandate has its roots in the behaviorism of the 1920s, when John B. Watson encouraged mothers not to "spoil" their children with affection. While we rightly recognize the foolishness of much of his advice, pieces of it remain.

Other cultures that do not have this philosophical baggage consider some of our child-rearing tactics to be bizarre, and even cruel. Kids with easygoing temperaments can often adapt to our rigid approach. But as you probably already know, children with spirited temperaments or ADHD do not. We need to retrain ourselves to think of our children's dependency needs as legitimate, and not as attempts to manipulate us or "get away" with something. As I noted in the sidebar earlier in this chapter, children whose dependency needs have been met are generally more securely attached to their parents, and cry less than children who've been forced to "behave."

Get Support

I've said it throughout this book, and I'll say it again: If you have a child with a behavioral concern, it can be very reassuring to talk to another parent who is struggling with the same issues. When you meet other parents whose children are acting the same way, it will be easier for you to believe that you are not the cause.

Children with behavioral issues can bring out the worst in their parents and teachers. Support is absolutely essential if you feel that you are losing control. These children are at very high risk of being abused, and to be truthful, it's not hard to see why. It is important that you find a person or group who will let you air your feelings in a safe way so that you do not take them out on your child.

Don't Make Any Permanent Decisions on Future Children Yet

In *Parenting the Fussy Baby and the High-Need Child* (1996), William and Martha Sears caution parents not to take any permanent steps to limit the size of their families until things are on a more even keel. They describe how parents in their practice had sometimes decided to get a vasectomy or tubal ligation, only to have their children grow out of their difficult stage. These parents often regretted their decision. If possible, wait until things settle down before making any permanent decision.

Conclusion

Mothering a child who has behavioral issues can quickly swamp your coping abilities and bring you to your emotional knees. You might feel overwhelmed and totally alone. If you do, take heart. There are others who have gone before you and will show you the way. Take advantage of some of the resources listed at the end of this chapter and find the solution that works best for you.

For Further Reading

Reading the stories of other parents struggling with similar concerns can be very reassuring. These books and Web sites can offer lots of assistance with any issue you are facing.

Resources for Temperament and ADHD

If you've never read a book about some of the issues you might be facing, these books are a great place to start. These are the ones that get passed from parent to parent. Each offers its own comforting advice.

Greene, R. 1998. *The Explosive Child*. New York: HarperCollins.
Kitzinger, S. 1990. *The Crying Baby*. New York: Penguin.
Kurcinka, M. S. 1991. *Raising Your Spirited Child*. New York: Harper Perennial.
Sears, W., and M. Sears. 1996. *Parenting the Fussy Baby and High-Need Child*. New York: Little, Brown.

Sears, W., and L. Thompson. 1998. *The A.D.D. Book: New Understandings, New Approaches to Parenting Your Child.* New York: Little, Brown.

ADD Consultations: www.addconsults.com

ADDvance: www.ADDvance.com. For women and girls with ADHD.

ADD Warehouse : www.addwarehouse.com or 800-233-9273.

AHDH News: www.adhdnews.com

Children and Adults with ADHD: www.chadd.org

Postpartum Education for Parents: www.sbpep.org

University of Illinois Extension: search for "Nibbles," then "Coping with the 'Spirited Child'": www.urbanext.uiuc.edu

Books on Anger and Parenting/ Positive Discipline Strategies

Kurcinka, M. S. 2000. *Kids, Parents, and Power Struggles: Winning for a Lifetime.* New York: HarperCollins.

McKay, M., et al. 1996. *When Anger Hurts Your Kids: A Parents' Guide.* Oakland, Calif.: New Harbinger.

Nelsen, J., C. Erwin, and C. Delzer. 1994. *Positive Discipline for Single Parents: A Practical Guide to Raising Children Who Are Responsible, Respectful, and Resourceful.* Rocklin, Calif.: Prima Publishing.

Samalin, N. 1991. *Love and Anger.* New York: Penguin.

Sears, W., and M. Sears. 1995. *The Discipline Book.* New York: Little, Brown.

CHAPTER 10

CHALLENGING CHILD II
MOTHERING A CHILD WITH HEALTH ISSUES

For Mary, each day begins early, as she must allow an extra two hours to get her daughter ready for school. Her days and weeks are filled with doctors' appointments, physical therapy, meeting with school personnel, and intense daily care of her child. By the end of the day, she is exhausted. She sometimes wishes she had more help, but she is also inspired by her daughter's gentle spirit and quiet dignity.

Mothering a child with a chronic illness or disability can be relentless and overwhelming. It can also be a source of personal growth and satisfaction. Your experience may contain elements of both. In this chapter, I describe some of the challenges of mothering a child with health concerns. Though there are a great number of health conditions that could be included in this chapter, I've focused on two broad categories: prematurity and chronic illness/disability.

Prematurity

Each year, more than 400,000 premature or low birth-weight babies are born. Fortunately, most of these babies now survive. However, babies born very early or very small are still at risk for a number of serious complications, including brain hemorrhages, chronic lung disease, respiratory distress, blindness or visual impairment, cerebral palsy, and language delays (American Association for Premature Infants 2000).

A premature birth is almost always a surprise. Mothers and fathers are often overwhelmed by the emergency nature of the birth. The neonatal intensive care unit (NICU) can be intimidating. Today, NICU personnel are much better about involving mothers and helping them cope with the psychological fallout of having a baby born too soon. But your baby may have been born before these changes were in place. Or you may have encountered a hospital staff that didn't seem to give you much attention, even recently.

Today's cost-consciousness in healthcare also contributes to the challenges new mothers face. Healthcare providers are being forced to reduce hospital stays, so many fragile babies are being released from the hospital with little help and support for mothers. According to the American Association for Premature Infants, premature babies are "falling through the cracks" of our healthcare system. Many parents cannot find the services they need for their children, including occupational, physical, and speech therapy.

Mothers of premature babies are often anxious for the health and well-being of their babies. And this anxiety can last long past the child's infancy. Sandy told me that she had been a very tiny premature baby at birth. As she was preparing to graduate from college with high honors, her mother said to her, "You're really okay, aren't you?" Sandy related the story with some exasperation, but it gives a glimpse into the fears and concerns her mother had. It was as if her mother had been holding her breath all these years, waiting to see if her child would be okay. Sandy's mother's reaction was not unusual. Linda, whose son was born at twenty-seven weeks and weighed two pounds, describes similar feelings:

> When my son was about sixteen months old, I began to have anxiety attacks. I don't think I ever dealt with all of the pain and heartache of the NICU. No matter how old or big our babies get, they will always be preemies to us.

Similar reactions have been noted in research studies, where mothers of preterm infants were found to feel less confident in their ability to parent than did mothers of full-term infants, particularly if they had been denied contact with their babies. They also had difficulties learning to read their babies' cues, and were less likely to hold them, make eye contact, or smile. These problems vanished, or at least diminished, when mothers had access to their babies and were given help and support (Kendall-Tackett with Kantor 1993). Patricia describes what it was like for her to give birth to a very ill premature baby:

My first child was born at thirty-five weeks with severe hyaline membrane disease. He was in the hospital for five months: in the NICU for four months and in intermediate care for one month. The depression started around the time he was three or four weeks old. Up until that time, everything had been so urgent. He had had a couple of arrests. It was overwhelming. Suddenly my son was doing better. Why was I feeling so bad? I had difficulties going to sleep. I was up several times during the night. It was difficult to wake up in the morning. I didn't want to do anything during the day except sleep and call the NICU to check in. I started to not eat well. I felt an impending sense of doom.

Your feelings after having a premature baby can be influenced by how early or sick your baby was at birth. They can also be influenced by your birth experience, how you were treated at the hospital, and how much support you had once your baby was released.

Level of Prematurity and Illness

If a baby was very premature (less than thirty weeks), very small (less than 1,500 grams), or very ill, you are more likely to be troubled than if your baby was healthy, relatively large, or only a couple of weeks early. Some babies, even if they are not very premature, have physical problems, including immature lungs, cerebral palsy, or intraventricular hemorrhage. Even babies who are not gravely ill may seem fragile and small. Not surprisingly, Blumberg (1980) found that the sicker the baby, the more depressed the mother.

Circumstances of the Birth

Your baby's birth may have occurred under emergency conditions. You may have sustained an injury, such as a car accident or physical assault, that brought on premature labor. A complication of pregnancy, such as a placenta previa, may have necessitated an emergency delivery. You may have been away from home when you went into labor, only to have your baby in an ambulance, cab, or emergency room away from your own doctor and family. Being separated from your baby may also have been traumatic. Your baby may have been taken away before you could even hold her, as Helen describes:

They took her away right after delivery. I never got to hold her. They brought her back, but my arms were tied to the delivery table. I wish they had released at least one arm. Leaving the hospital without the baby was really bad. I left early because I didn't want to leave at 11 A.M. with all the other moms and babies.

The Medical Situation

While care of babies in NICUs has much improved, you may have had your baby at a time when parents were excluded. Watching the staff perform medical interventions can also be very difficult. For Jan, the worst part was watching them put a tube down her baby's throat. She could hear her baby cry and gag, and couldn't do anything about it. Even several years later, thinking about it makes her cry: "I shouldn't complain because she only had a few preemie problems. Others in the nursery were so sick. But it was very stressful."

Medical personnel may have also been insensitive, and made comments that were hurtful or rude. Patricia described how the majority of doctors and nurses caring for her son were great. But even after ten years, there was one comment that still rankles:

A second-year resident said the worst thing to me. He said, "You see that baby over there? We called the parents" (which meant that the baby was going to die), "but your baby is the sickest one on the unit." He was implying that our baby was sicker than the one who was going to die.

Anticipatory Grieving

Anticipatory grieving is another common reaction, that can present some challenges for you. As you became convinced that your baby would not survive, you may have started to distance yourself from him in order to prepare for his eventual death. When your baby recovered and lived, your mourning was interrupted, and you had to readjust your focus. Having come so close to death, it may have taken some time for you to assimilate the reality that your baby would live.

The Transition to Home

The transition to home can be difficult for parents, especially after a lengthy hospital stay. Premature babies often act differently than full-term babies their same age. They are often more sensitive to stimulation and easily become overwhelmed. When babies withdraw, mothers may think their babies are rejecting them. Sometimes, mothers respond by withdrawing from their babies. This seems especially true in cases where the baby is very sick, as was demonstrated in one research study (Jarvis et al. 1989). In this study researchers compared three groups of premature babies: those with no medical complications, those who were moderately ill (respiratory distress syndrome), and those who were very ill (bronchopulmonary dysplasia) at four and eight months of age. As predicted, degree of illness did influence the mother/infant interaction at both time points. Mothers of the sickest infants emotionally withdrew and became less responsive to them over time. But mothers of moderately ill babies actually became more responsive over time.

Continuing health problems may have made your transition home more difficult too. Although your baby was well enough to be released from the hospital, she was still not "well." You may have had to scramble for services your baby needed. Andrea describes how medical mismanagement and her son's continuing illness filled her with anxiety:

> In his discharge conference, the pediatrician proposed that there may be something else going on. She thought maybe it was cystic fibrosis. I went crazy waiting for the results. She also tested for gammaglobulin, but never contacted us about the results. I assumed no news was good news. He was sick constantly the first year and a half. I found out the report on the gammaglobulin had been positive. No one did anything. He could have died. It was a nightmare.

Having been premature, your child is more vulnerable to chronic illness and disability. For many mothers with premature infants, this is "phase two" in the story of their children's health problems. But there are many other mothers and children whose stories begin here. In the next section, I describe some of the challenges that mothers of children with chronic conditions face.

Chronic Illness and Disability

Myriad illnesses affect children. Common chronic childhood illnesses include asthma, diabetes, and autoimmune diseases such as juvenile rheumatoid arthritis and ulcerative colitis. Childhood cancer, once almost always fatal, is now being survived by many of the children who get it, and is considered a chronic illness rather than a fatal disease.

"Disability" also covers a wide range of conditions. There are sensory disabilities such as blindness and deafness, motor impairments such as cerebral palsy, and developmental disorders including mental retardation, autism, pervasive developmental disorder (PDD), and Asperger syndrome. There are emotional disabilities such as depression and post-traumatic stress disorder. Even learning disabilities and ADHD can be included in the list.

There is substantial overlap between the conditions described in this and the previous chapter. For example, a child who was born prematurely is at increased risk for cerebral palsy, ADHD, and learning disabilities. Some 20 percent of children with learning disabilities may also have ADHD. Also, current thinking about developmental disorders places ADHD on the same continuum as PDD, autism, and Asperger syndrome, although it is important to stress that ADHD will not progress to one of these more serious illnesses.

Mothers are often the ones who feel the full brunt of their children's health issues. In one recent study of parents in the year following the birth of a child with a congenital abnormality, mothers were significantly more likely to report personal strain than were fathers (Hunfeld et al. 1999). A child with a chronic health condition can strain family finances, stress relationships, and cut families off from important sources of support (LaPlante et al. 1996).

Some parents are so overwhelmed that they do the unthinkable—abuse their children. Sullivan and Knutson (2000) studied more than 50,000 children in the Midwest. They found that children with disabilities were three times more likely to be neglected and physically, emotionally, or sexually abused compared with children who do not have disabilities. Except for sexual abuse, most of the abuse occurred within the family and mothers were the abusers in 67 percent of the cases.

If you are struggling, it is important for you to recognize that you might respond to overwhelming stress by maltreating your child. While most mothers have occasional angry feelings, you must find help and support so that you do not vent them on your child.

Certain factors influence how mothers feel in response to a child with health concerns, even when those illnesses and disabilities differ from one another. These factors will influence how challenging your child's condition is for you.

Seriousness of Health Concern

The higher the degree of risk for your baby or child, the more challenging a health concern will be for you. During the course of a life-threatening event, you might find that everything else goes on hold. Your life is reduced to day-to-day, or even hour-to-hour, functioning.

If your child's condition is serious but not life-threatening, you may still have many of the same concerns. Depending on how much help your child needs with the activities of daily living, and whether she spends time at school or is home all day, your days may be filled with caring for your child and transporting her to and from appointments with physical or occupational therapists, doctors, and other healthcare providers.

Obviousness or Stigma of Impairment

The type and obviousness of your child's impairment can influence how others react to you and your child, and also how you feel about yourself and your child. It might seem odd, but there is a hierarchy of acceptability of illness and disability. Some chronic conditions are more likely to engender sympathy and support than others. In summarizing the research literature, psychologist Rhoda Olkin (1999) notes that our judgments are influenced by the severity, visibility, and treatability of the condition; its effect on life expectancy; and whether the condition is perceived as contagious. In the hierarchy, conditions such as asthma or diabetes are not obvious, and therefore more acceptable. Conditions that are more obvious are less acceptable and more stigmatized. Olkin indicates that the most highly stigmatized conditions are para- and quadriplegia, multiple sclerosis, cerebral palsy, and facial disfigurement.

In trying to explain why these stigmas exist, Olkin notes that all of us have ideas about how the body should appear, move, function, think, behave, and communicate. When people deviate from these standards, we stigmatize them. The more people deviate, the greater the level of stigma (Olkin 1999). Even when there are no particular health consequences to an impairment, people may still shun your child if he or she looks different than other people.

Strenuousness of Managing the Condition

Some conditions require little effort from caretakers, while others require a great deal. The more strenuous the caretaking regimen, the more challenging it will be for you. For example, mothers of children with dietary restrictions must plan and be vigilant every day. Children with peanut allergies can die from eating anything with peanuts, so their mothers may have to go to great lengths to ensure that their children are not exposed. Indeed, at mothers' insistence some school districts have even gone so far as to request that all parents avoid the use of peanut butter if a child with a peanut allergy goes to a school. Another illness with dietary restrictions is diabetes: eating a forbidden food can bring on a coma or even death. Parents of a diabetic child must monitor the child's blood sugar levels and supervise his insulin injections. Managing this illness is a daily event.

Another type of condition that involves frequent management is orthopedic impairment, which may require daily exercises to strengthen muscles and protect joints. In addition, these exercises may need to be regularly supervised by a professional, such as an occupational or physical therapist.

Children in wheelchairs may also need a great deal of assistance in the activities of daily living, such as dressing, bathing, and toileting. Normal morning routines will tend to take longer so mothers will need to allow extra time for almost all activities. As children grow, managing these activities may become physically strenuous as well.

Beliefs about Why It Occurred

According to Gerry Koocher (2000), chief psychologist at Children's Hospital in Boston, parents may be either aided or hindered in coping with their children's illnesses by their beliefs about why it occurred. If parents believe they are responsible or that God is punishing them by making their children ill, coping will be much more difficult. On the other hand, if they believe that their children's conditions have also brought some positives, they are in a better position to cope, as Elena describes:

> When I questioned why this terrible thing was happening, I kept in mind Billy's strong spirit and that something larger than myself was taking place. I thanked him for coming into our lives, and always felt pride at everything he accomplished and fought for. I am constantly amazed at the blessing of his presence in my life, what a gift it is to live this life in his company, as his mother.

Attempting to understand why something occurred is a natural part of coming to terms with a difficult event. However, when seeking a reason turns to guilt and blame, it ceases to be a helpful strategy for coping.

Suddenness

Illness or disability can come suddenly, with no warning. In *Healing the Child* (1996), Nancy Cain describes how her son became critically ill after being exposed to *E. coli* bacteria. He went from bright and healthy to deathly ill almost overnight. After he recovered from his infection, he developed seizures that were often life-threatening. This family's world was forever changed by their son's illness. Having no warning of these impending changes can make it more difficult to cope.

Cumulative Stressors

Families may be faced with multiple stressors at the same time, all contributing to a higher level of overall stress. Some types of stressors you may experience as the parent of an ill or disabled child include financial problems, strained relationships with your partner or other family members, single parenting, job pressures, and lack of support. Not surprisingly, the total number of children in a family can make a difference in the mother's stress level. Mothers are more able to cope with a child with health issues if they have only one child. Children with health issues born later into the family can be a greater source of stress because mothers have other children to care for as well.

Some Common Feelings

Parenting a child with a health concern tends to bring up certain feelings. I discuss some of the most common reactions below. It is important that you recognize and acknowledge your feelings, but it is also important that you get the help you need. According to Olkin (1999), there are two important tasks for parents of a child with a disability: accepting your child as a full member of the family, and accepting the disability itself. These tasks will be easier for you if you are not struggling to take care of everything all by yourself.

Resentment and Anger

Resentment is a common feeling among parents whose children have health issues. If you have a child who is sick or has a disability, you may resent the changes you've had to make in your life. You may have had to quit your job. Outside activities may have been curtailed indefinitely. Your family may have needed to move to be closer to a medical facility. Having a medically fragile child may strain your finances to the limit.

You might also find that you are angry with others. If you are married, having a child with an illness or disability can strain your marriage. In fact, many marriages do not survive. If you have other, healthy children, you may resent their demands on your time, or even that they are healthy when your other child is sick.

The constant need to navigate the medical or educational systems may leave you feeling frustrated and angry much of the time. You may be mad at other mothers who just don't "get it." You may be mad at society because of its marginalization of families of children with special needs. And you may be mad at God for allowing this to happen to you and your family.

Guilt

Guilt is also common among mothers of children with disabilities or illnesses. Many mothers wonder if they somehow "caused" the problems their children are experiencing. Guilt may also come from your healthcare providers. Unfortunately, as the healthcare industry becomes more cost-conscious, you may find yourself feeling guilty for having a child that costs your insurer more. Many parents have related stories of being pressured into prenatal testing, and into terminating a pregnancy when an anomaly was identified. If you chose not to have the testing, or not to terminate the pregnancy, you might feel guilty for bringing a less-than-perfect child into the world. Even if you feel positive about your decision, others may question you and act horrified that you would "purposely" have a child with an abnormality. Not surprisingly, this is an issue of concern among many in the disability-rights community.

You may feel guilty for not being able to meet everyone's needs, or about spending time away from your partner and other children. Finally, you may feel guilty for failing to live up to expectations of yourself or others to be a perfect mother. According to Miriam Greenspan (1998), mothers are often pressured into silence about the difficulties of caring for children with disabilities. According to her, anything other than serenity and acceptance indicates that you still have "unresolved feelings" about your child's disability:

> Many mothers of children with disabilities prefer to keep their pain and exhaustion private, not wanting to fuel the argument that children with disabilities are a "burden" to their parents and to society. This is a self-enforced silencing that is part of what it means to be "marginalized." (43)

If the job of mother often feels impossible for mothers of well children, it feels doubly so for mothers of children with special needs. And as with any type of mothering, there will be good and bad days. To indicate that it is possible to get to a place of total acceptance, where things never bother you, is unrealistic and places an unfair burden on you.

Isolation

Isolation is another fact of life for families of children with health concerns. Other mothers may discourage their children from playing with your child, because your child's condition makes them uncomfortable. You might find that you are no longer invited to functions as a family.

When talking with other mothers, you may find that the concerns they express seem minor compared to your experiences. This may increase your sense that others have no idea what you are going through. How in the world can you describe the relentless nature of your caregiving responsibilities? Or discuss feeding using a gastric tube, the daily care of an ostomy, or how to correctly fasten a leg brace? How do you explain that exposure to a "normal" childhood illness like chicken pox can have life-threatening consequences for your child? Margaret withdrew from volunteer work that she enjoyed because her son was "out of control" at meetings:

> My son has been assessed hyperlexic and diagnosed autistic, and has a secondary diagnosis of ADHD. Before we made dietary changes (he is now casein- and gluten-free as per *Special Diets for Special Kids* by Lisa Lewis), he was either going to sleep around 1 A.M. or getting up and staying awake running around in the night for a few hours. He sleeps regularly now unless he gets gluten, casein, or a Snickers bar. Chocolate once kept him awake for twenty-four hours. And me? After toughing it out with another special-needs child we lost in 1992 (Brian had leu-

kemia from three until his death at three months short of thirteen), I am finally headed to my doctor to ask for some antianxiety medication.

Another isolating aspect of caring for children with special needs is the reaction (or lack of a reaction) of others in the wake of a life-threatening complication or episode. If your family has suffered a medical crisis, you may be taken aback by the sudden awareness that the world has continued on as before. You feel that the outside world does not acknowledge the dramatic change in your life. This type of experience further indicates the uniqueness of your situation.

Uncertainty

Your uncertainty can start with your knowing something is wrong but not having any explanation. A correct diagnosis may be months or even years in the making. The condition you are trying to name may be elusive, with symptoms that come and go, and tests that come back as "inconclusive." Your child may receive several different diagnoses before actually finding one that fits.

Uncertainty also involves looking into the future and wondering what it will bring. Will she be the object of ridicule? Will he be able to get the services he needs? Will she be able to graduate from high school or college? Will she ever get married and have a family? What kind of life will he have? Will tomorrow bring a decline in functioning? Will she die? What will happen to him after you die?

Depression and Burnout

You may be so fatigued and burned out, that you lose touch with others and sink into depression or despair. Give yourself permission to acknowledge what you have accomplished just by living your life. But also remember that you cannot do it alone. Everyone needs occasional nurturing—including you.

Sadness and Loss

Related to depression is sadness associated with the death of the "dream" child. Depending on the type and severity of the disability or condition, you may have to scale back your expectations about what your child will be able to do. Most of us start off wanting our children to be healthy, smart, athletic, attractive, and popular—even if we, ourselves, don't have these characteristics. As your child matures, there will be many times when you realize that your child is outside the norm. And this may make you feel sad.

Recently, I attended a session for parents of special-needs children held at a conference for breastfeeding families. One of the more poignant moments was when these mothers acknowledged that a dream had died: the dream that if you breastfeed your baby, everything will be great. These women had breastfed their babies, yet all of them had serious conditions.

Potential for Joy

The feelings I've discussed above help identify some of the challenges that parents of children with health concerns face. I wanted to voice and validate these feelings. But I don't want to leave you with the impression that this is the whole story. Parents of children with special needs acknowledge the difficulties but also point to many positives.

For example, many of these children demonstrate great compassion for others. Having a disability or chronic condition can mature children beyond their years. As adults, they may reach out to other families with children who are like them. Miriam Greenspan (1998) described how her daughter would suddenly display flashes of insight about people that would take her breath away. Where, she would wonder, did her then six-year-old daughter learn *that*?

Parents themselves learn many things. Mothers often become extremely knowledgeable about whatever condition their children have. In some cases, they know as much as or even more than many of their children's doctors. Some, like the mother-activists described in chapter 4, have lobbied for changes that have affected hundreds or even thousands of other families with special needs.

Parents of children with health concerns often mention how they have become much more patient than they used to be. Having been through real crises, they are less likely to get rattled by events that would have bothered them earlier, or that bother other parents. These parents have learned to focus on what's important rather than being so distracted by the cares of this world. In many cases, they've streamlined their lives and have achieved a level of simplicity others would like to imitate. Children with special needs can also display a grace that transcends their physical limitations, as Miriam Greenspan describes:

Esther herself is the best source of whatever courage and resistance I muster in the challenge of mothering her. She has taught me acceptance and gratitude for each moment in a way that has brought a very special kind of joy into my life. If there is a nightmare here, it is my fear that the world, when I leave it, will not be sufficient to hold her or to see her truly. The unanswered question is: Will her gifts find their place in a world not yet worthy of her, or of any of our children? (58–59)

In writing about disability, psychologist Rhoda Olkin (1999) describes how the research literature is often very one-sided in its presentation of families with children with disabilities. The studies emphasize the "burdens" of taking care of these children but rarely discuss the positive aspects. While we must be realistic about the difficulties that families encounter, and ensure that they get the help and support they need, we must also not adopt the attitude that these children are not "worth it" and that they only bring negative things to their families.

What You Can Do

Fortunately, there are some concrete things you can do to help break the isolation and ease the strain of mothering a child with a health concern. Perhaps the most important message I can give is that you are not alone.

Become an Expert on Your Child's Condition

As I suggested in the previous chapter, dedicate yourself to learning (or keep learning) everything about your child's condition. You and your partner are the ones who will have to advocate for your child through the educational and medical systems.

The information you gather is not only helpful in working with doctors and schools, but it is helpful for you as well. Children with health concerns often act differently than children who do not have these issues. By understanding their needs and limitations, you can start anticipating situations where they are likely to have difficulties. This can help you prevent some recurring problems that you encounter.

Join with Others and Get Support

In order to break free of isolation, you must find other parents who have had similar experiences. Fortunately, groups for almost any condition abound. And don't forget online support. There are chatrooms and LISTSERVs available on almost any subject. With these, you can access support twenty-four hours a day. This can be a boon for parents who are isolated geographically or who cannot get to a support group. Just reading the posts of other parents will let you know that you are not alone. You may also find that other parents are some of the best sources of information on what works and what doesn't.

When using any of these resources, however, one caution is in order. Sometimes support groups can be counterproductive if they are overly negative and interested more in complaining than in trying to do something constructive. While you must feel free to air some of your most negative feelings, too much time spent dwelling on the negative aspects of your situation can make it worse. If you find that you are walking away from sessions of support feeling worse than when you came in, it's probably time to look for another group.

Continue to Nurture Relationships with Others

Parenting children with health concerns may leave you with little time for other relationships. You may feel so intent on meeting the needs of your child that you neglect the needs of your partner, family members, and friends. These people may seem like one more group that needs you, but you shouldn't forget that you need them too. Having healthy, reciprocal relationships with others is a great buffer against all kinds of stress. While nurturing you relationships may feel like one more thing to add to your endless list, think of it as self-care.

But sometimes, the people closest to you say the most hurtful things. In their efforts to come to terms with what has happened to your child, other family members may try to assign blame for his or her condition. They may speculate about whether your family was the source of the "faulty genes," or whether you worked too much while you were pregnant. They may also be the ones to offer unsolicited child-rearing advice. In these situations, remember that you have a right to get the kind of help and support you need. If people make hurtful remarks, gently let them know that that kind of comment is hurtful and does not help. If they persist, you may have to distance yourself from that relationship.

Help Your Other Children Cope

Sometimes, your other children will feel pushed aside because it seems that all your energy is focused on caring for the child with a chronic condition. Their reaction is understandable, but everyone in the family will be happier if you make time for your other children as well. That may mean turning the care of your child with a chronic condition over to someone else for a while. Recognize that your other children may also resent how their sibling's difficulties impact them. They may feel embarrassed by the way their sibling acts in public, or the stares they get. Your other children must also have a safe place to vent without harming the child with difficulties.

Even young children can be involved in caring and watching out for the needs of your child with health concerns. Their experiences with their brother or sister may also make them more sensitive to the needs of others, and may even encourage their entry into the healthcare field as adults. While you do want to involve your other children, you must also be careful to let them be kids as well. You might also want to encourage them to develop relationships in your extended family or with other adults so that they will have plenty of adult time too.

Learn How Much Information to Share

When dealing with any family issue that is outside the norm, you need to learn—usually through trial and error—how much information you should share with others. Sometimes, we mothers offer way too much explanation, usually in an apologetic way. On the other hand, a forthright, nondefensive request for the help your child needs can go a long way. For example, you might explain to the mother of a classmate that your child can't go to her house to play because the environment may not be accessible for your child, but that you would be happy to have her child over to play at your house.

I have learned to be forthright in asking for accommodations I need instead of assuming that others "should" know. Most people understand, and are happy to do what I ask. But there are still people who don't, and who actually give me a hard time about making necessary accommodations and even about my using a handicapped tag for my car. While it would be nice if everyone were responsive, it's not always possible. In time, you will learn whom you can really share with and who would rather not hear it. It's also helpful to practice some nondefensive answers like "that's what works best for our family." As you gain confidence, you'll feel more comfortable with getting what you need without feeling it is necessary to explain your situation to people who refuse to understand.

By acknowledging your challenges, and reaching out to others for help and support, you also become ready to embrace the positives that come with mothering a child with special needs. In closing, I'd like to share the words of Amy, the mother of a boy with Asperger syndrome:

> Accepting your challenged child requires that you go through a grief process. You must mourn, in a sense, your vision of the child you expected your precious baby to become. Only then can you move on to accept the child you have been given. Eventually you will be able to look beyond your child's limitations and celebrate his or her uniqueness.

For Further Reading

Here are some of the best of the many books available for parents of children with health concerns. You should also contact some of the online sources for information about specific conditions.

Resources for Parents of Children with Health Concerns

Cain, N. 1996. *Healing the Child: A Mother's Story.* New York: Rawson Associates.

Finston, P. 1992. *Parenting Plus: Raising Children with Special Health Needs.* New York: Viking Penguin.

Gordon, S. 1993. *One Miracle at a Time: Getting Help for a Child with a Disability.* New York: Simon & Schuster.

Klaus, M. H., P. H. Klaus, and J. H. Kennell. 1996. *Bonding: Building the Foundations of Secure Attachment and Independence.* Cambridge, Mass.: Perseus Publishing.

Naseef, R. 1997. *Special Children, Challenged Parents.* Secaucus, N.J.: Carol Publishing Group.

Sears, W., and M. Sears. 1995. *The Discipline Book.* New York: Little, Brown. See especially the chapter on parenting a child with special needs.

Preemies

ABC's of parenting: Find links to other premature baby sites at www.abcparenting.com

Early Arrivals: for preemie supplies go to www.earlyarrivals.com

The Early Edition: an online newsletter for parents of preemies at www.home.vicnet.net.au/~earlyed

KidsHealth: Search for "primer on preemies" at www.kidshealth.org

Disability/Health Issues

Association for the Care of Children's Health: www.acch.org

Children with Disabilities: www.childrenwithdisabilities.ncjrs.org

Federation for Children with Special Needs: www.fcsn.org

National Information Center for Children and Youth with Disabilities: www.nichcy.org

CHAPTER 11

HELLO-GOODBYE
MOTHERING AND CHILDBEARING LOSS

> In a moment's time, our world shatters like fine china. And the darkness comes. For some, it was a phone call from the doctor. Still others were all alone. Perhaps you found your precious baby lifeless in the crib, a heartbeat suddenly stopped. Or maybe, like me, it was in a cold, dark room that you felt life slip away as you watched a black, silent ultrasound. Our stories are all different, but our pain is the same. (Linda DeYmaz 1996, 1)

Childbearing loss is one of the greatest challenges mothers can face. Yet it is far more common than you might believe. Some estimate that over one-third of babies conceived each year in the United States do not survive (Panuthos and Romeo 1984). You may have lost your child through miscarriage, stillbirth, prematurity and neonatal death, or sudden infant death syndrome (SIDS). There may have been an accident at birth or a chromosomal anomaly. Your baby may have contracted a fatal infection.

You may wonder how you can go on after your precious baby has died. No matter how devastating your loss or deep your sorrow, there is hope for healing. In their poignant book *Ended Beginnings* (1984), Claudia Panuthos and Cathy Romeo describe the process this way:

> There are no shortcuts or quick fixes in these phases of healing, for grief is relentless, and it will not be shortchanged. We cannot completely evade its presence in our lives no matter how desperately we may try. Yet peace

is possible in the mind and the heart when grief and pain are embraced, released and openly expressed. (xvi)

Types of Childbearing Loss

Loss is no respecter of persons. Women of all nationalities and income levels have suffered from childbearing losses. Some of you have experienced one type, while others have experienced two, three, or even more. Years of infertility treatments may have finally resulted in a pregnancy that ended in miscarriage. You may have had a baby born so early that he could not survive, or lost a baby to SIDS only to miscarry on a subsequent pregnancy. The pain from each of these experiences is real. In this section, I describe some of the more common types of childbearing loss. Although the focus of this chapter is pregnancy and infant loss (for these are the most common types), much of what I share in this chapter can apply to the death of an older child as well.

Miscarriage

Each year, there are an estimated 600,000 to 800,000 women who miscarry in the United States, and these numbers probably underestimate the true incidence. Miscarriage is the most common and least acknowledged form of infant loss. It is often experienced in private, leaving you to grieve alone.

Some women seem to take miscarriage in stride, and are ready to "try again" in relatively short order. Many other women, however, feel a deep sense of loss after a miscarriage. A problem arises when people in your life assume that you have taken this event "in stride" and are then surprised by your sense of loss.

The physical aspects of miscarriage can also be traumatic. Your first hint that you were about to lose your baby may have been a small amount of blood. You may have frantically called your doctor's office only to be told there was little that you could do. Or they may have told you that "spotting" is normal for many pregnancies. Spotting might have continued for several days, as you agonized over whether you would lose this pregnancy.

Rather than a little blood, there may have been a lot, either gradually or suddenly. Gushing blood and passing large clots are frightening, and in the case of miscarriage, they are harbingers of impending loss. Bleeding may have accompanied painful contractions that surprised you with their intensity.

Many women find the aftermath of miscarriage to be one of the most traumatic parts. It may have occurred at home, or on a gurney in the emergency room. Hospital staff may have treated you in a callous or cavalier way. You may have found out that your baby was gone by looking at a black ultrasound screen.

You may have had to undergo a D & C to make sure that there were no remnants of your pregnancy left behind. These surgical procedures can be frightening and painful, and can reinforce your feelings of powerlessness. Even if the staff is kind, it does not completely take away from the invasive nature of these procedures.

The psychological and emotional impact of miscarriage is compounded for women who have had more than one. Your pregnancies may have been kept secret, meaning that you suffer alone when you miscarry. Each subsequent pregnancy is filled with fear, as you wonder if this one will last. Kathleen Diamond (1991) describes her experience of multiple miscarriage this way:

> The mourning process became shorter after each miscarriage, because I was resigned to failure and did not actually think each pregnancy was real. After each miscarriage, I went about business as usual. No one else could possibly feel as badly as I did, and besides, I had a sense of terrible shame and failure. (67)

Miscarriage might also occur in the midst of treatment for infertility. You may have endured months of hormone treatments, invasive exams, and daily temperature charts. Your pregnancy may have been the result of one or more sessions of in vitro fertilization. With each miscarriage, your odds for having a baby seemed to lessen, leaving you with an overwhelming sense of hopelessness. Getting and staying pregnant may have become the driving force of your life.

Whether you have had one or many miscarriages, you will find that there are few outlets for you to acknowledge your grief. You have probably had to mourn these loses alone (Panuthos and Romeo 1984).

Infertility

Related to miscarriage is another form of childbearing loss: infertility. Infertility is also relatively common. In the 1995 National Survey of Family Growth, more than 6 million women reported "impaired fecundity": difficulty in conceiving or carrying a child to term (Fidler and Bernstein 1999). This is approximately 10 percent of women ages fifteen to forty-four. It is not unusual for women to have experienced miscarriage, sometimes several times, before, during, and after treatment for infertility. Indeed, some health programs won't even start a work-up for infertility until a woman has had her third miscarriage.

Infertility brings with it its own emotional repercussions. First of all, it interferes with a fundamental and highly valued human need. Fidler and Bernstein (1999) liken its emotional impact to that of cancer or heart disease. Some of the negative effects of infertility include isolation, depression, reduced job performance, and lower life satisfaction. Testing and treatment for infertility can consume your life. The testing is invasive, expensive, and often painful. The most intimate details of your life are laid bare. Sex loses its spontaneity and becomes mechanical. The onset of each period brings the realization that you are once again not pregnant. You may begin to wonder why this is happening to you when women who do not want children seem to get pregnant with ease.

There are also physical consequences of infertility that relate to childbearing losses. Women undergoing treatment for infertility are often given ovulation-enhancing drugs, which dramatically increase the likelihood of multiple births. Multiples are more likely to have any number of health concerns, including prematurity and low birth weight. The danger of death dramatically increases, especially for higher order multiples (triplets and more). The mortality rate for these babies is fifteen times greater than it is for singletons (Kiely et al. 1992). You may find that you are faced with the challenge of mothering your surviving baby or babies while mourning the loss of one or more.

Multiple embryos may also be a result of in vitro fertilization. To increase the likelihood of pregnancy, healthcare providers may implant several embryos. This raises ethical dilemmas that parents of previous generations never had to face. One issue is that of "selective reduction," where the number of fetuses is reduced since fewer fetuses have greater chances of survival. On the other hand, mothers working very hard to become and stay pregnant are often not receptive to the idea of terminating any of their pregnancies. Some countries, such as Great Britain, are now limiting the number of embryos that can be implanted at once to three, which may help to prevent this dilemma.

It's also important to recognize that not all treatment for infertility ends with the birth of a baby. Couples may endure years of testing, treatment, and miscarriages before coming to the conclusion that they are unable to have a biological child. This is also experienced as a significant loss. Even when mothers go on to adopt, they may feel marginalized, though their path to motherhood is no less heroic than that of other mothers. And often it is more so. Even after a woman becomes a mother through adoption, the sting of infertility may linger for years (Smith et al. 1998).

Stillbirth

Another form of childbearing loss is the death of a baby at or near term. This occurs in approximately 1 in 80 births, accounting for more than 195,000 deaths per year. Stillbirth has a variety of causes. It could be due to an accident involving the cord or placenta, an infection, or toxemia in the mother.

In some cases of stillbirth, the baby dies before labor begins. Mothers often have a sense that something is wrong. They may have felt no movement, or started to bleed and had sudden searing pains. Or there may have been no warning at all. You may have learned of your baby's death during a routine examination, when your doctor or midwife could not find a heartbeat.

Once you discovered that your baby was dead, you may have found yourself in the nightmarish scenario of needing to carry a dead baby for days or even weeks, awaiting labor. Unbelievably, you still needed to go through labor knowing that your baby would not be alive at the end. Since your baby was already dead, the staff may have given you strong pain medication, exacerbating your feeling that this was all happening to someone else.

Perhaps your baby died during labor. Things may have been going well, then suddenly the cord may have prolapsed, or the uterus ruptured. Your baby may have contracted an infection during labor. Some type of chromosomal abnormality may have only allowed your baby to live for a brief time after birth.

In some situations, your baby may have died because of the incompetence or negligence of the medical staff. They may have left you alone when you had a complication. They may have ignored your pleas for help, or misread the fetal monitor. This can be one of the most difficult deaths to accept because it might have been preventable. You may actually hate the people you feel are responsible, and even consider legal action.

Although your baby has died, your body may act like you have recently given birth to a living baby: your breasts fill with milk; you have lochia. Some mothers have described this experience as their whole body's weeping for the lost child.

Prematurity and Neonatal Death

Preterm birth (birth at less than thirty-seven completed weeks of gestation) is the second leading cause of infant mortality in the United States. Related to preterm birth is low birth weight (LBW), or having a birth weight that is less than five pounds or 2,500 grams. The babies at highest risk are those who are classified as "very low birth weight," or less than three and a half pounds or 1,500 grams. Approximately 7 percent of babies are of low birth weight, and approximately 1.5 percent are of very low birth weight. According to the Centers for Disease Control and Prevention, in 1997 65 percent of all infant deaths occurred among the 7.5 percent of infants born at low birth weight.

No one knows for certain what causes preterm birth, but some risk factors have been identified. Teen pregnancy, poverty, and lack of prenatal care all contribute to low birth weight. Premature/LBW babies are twice as likely to be born to mothers who smoke. The birth of a previous premature baby increases the risk that you will have another baby who is premature. Having multiples also increases the likelihood of both prematurity and LBW. African Americans have approximately twice as many LBW babies as their white counterparts, a disparity that can't be fully explained by independent risk factors such as poverty. But there are plenty of women who do not have any of these risk factors, and yet give birth to premature and low birth-weight babies. You may have agonized over whether you did anything that caused your baby to be premature.

Mothers of premature babies find that they are faced with dilemmas about how much intervention to allow. Babies born too early or too small probably cannot survive. Yet the line of "too early" is often blurry. Babies that are routinely saved today would have died even fifteen years ago. If your baby was born some time ago, you may face the realization that had your baby been born now, she may have survived.

You may have endured a week or a month (or longer) of wondering if your baby would survive, only to have him finally succumb. Your baby probably never left the hospital. He may have needed to be rushed from your side to an NICU that was far away, leaving you to drive many miles to be by your baby's side during your own recovery. You may have needed to stay in a city far from home, returning each night to an empty hotel room. None of your family or friends may have ever even seen your baby, increasing the feelings of unreality surrounding her birth and death.

Sudden Infant Death Syndrome (SIDS)

Sudden infant death syndrome (SIDS) is the unexplained death of a baby less than one year of age that remains unexplained even after an autopsy, examination of the death scene, and a review of the case history. Approximately 90 percent of SIDS deaths occur by six months of age. SIDS affects approximately 1 in 700 babies born in the U.S., but the rate is lower in other countries (Sears 1995). It is the third most common form of death for babies, according to the Centers for Disease Control and Prevention (1999).

While we have been able to identify some risk factors for SIDS, its cause remains a mystery. Babies who were exposed to cigarette smoke, were born prematurely, slept on their stomachs, or were formula-fed are at highest risk. However, there are many babies who have all these risk factors but do not succumb to SIDS. Conversely, some babies who have none of these risk factors do.

Mothers whose babies die of SIDS are usually overwhelmed by the suddenness of the loss. Babies have died on the day that they had a well-baby check. They have died at their mothers' breast, or while sleeping next to their mothers. In the next section, I share the story of one mother whose baby died of SIDS.

Jonathan's Song: One Mother's Story of SIDS

For Joan Valk, December 8, 1989 started like any day. But the events of that day forever changed her life. When Joan went to check on her baby Jonathan in his crib, she made the heart-stopping discovery that he was not breathing. Her neighbor made a frantic 911 call, and the baby was rushed to the hospital. An hour later, the doctor came out to tell Joan and her husband, Henk, that their baby was gone. Jonathan, her second son, died that day of SIDS. He was three months old.

> All I could think of was that I needed to be with Jonathan. I said: "I want to see him. I've got to be with him." The nurse said "Of course, of course." And they brought us into the room where my little baby lay, wrapped in a white sheet on the gurney.
>
> When I reached the stretcher on which he lay, I pulled the white sheet open, exposing his pale little body.

As I sobbed, "Oh, Jonathan, Jonathan, I loved you. I loved you so much." I caressed his naked body with my hand, touching every part, trying to etch into my mind what I soon would no longer be able to see. I looked up at Henk and he was weeping, tears streaming down his face, his head tipped back in disbelief. The nurses scurried to get chairs for both of us. I think they were afraid that one of us would faint. I covered Jonathan back up and picked him up to hold him. He had a tube sticking out of his mouth and a needle in his right shoulder. I asked the nurse if they could take them out, but she said no. As I held him, I stroked his coppery brown hair. I told the nurse that his hair had just started to grow in. Her eyes were red as she wept with us in our grief.

I turned to Henk and said, "What can we do? I can't just walk away and leave him here." The nurses assured us that we could stay as long as we wanted to, and just hold him and be with him. I pulled his little hand out from underneath the sheet and held his fingers and stroked them. I touched his toes and his feet. I looked and looked at his face and hair. Even with the tube and the discoloration around his eyes, he looked peaceful. I have always been afraid of death and dead bodies, but Jonathan did not frighten me. He was simply my son.

Henk took Jonathan out of my arms and I didn't know what he was going to do. I was afraid that he was taking him away from me. But he just wanted to pray. He committed our son back into the Lord's hands and thanked Him for the time we were able to have with Jonathan. Then he gave him back to me to hold. Before that I was afraid to let go of Jonathan. After that prayer, I felt that it was time to leave him and go home. The nurse came in and I handed Jonathan to her. I kissed the top of his head and touched him one last time. Then we left the room and stepped out into the corridor.

Everything after that is after. This is about Jonathan, and our story goes on. We said good-bye to him the best way we could and then tried to pick up the pieces. The great pain and emptiness are still quite real, but not as present every day. His name means "God's precious gift," and that's what we put on his tombstone, but I've come to realize that is what all children are. Children are precious, people are precious, each day is precious. That is what I learned from my son's short life and his death. We miss him so much. That will never fade. I know he is with my Father in heaven and that helps, but there are times when I just want to hold him one more time, nurse him one more time, touch him, hear him just one last time.

But every time I feel that loss, that great void, I also feel grateful for the time we were able to have with one very special little boy, who gave us great joy for an incredibly short time and who we will never forget. No bitter grief could ever poison that, the wonderful sweet time we had with our son Jonathan Gerhard Valk.

Some Common Reactions

Everyone grieves in a different way, and with a different intensity. Saul Bloom, a father whose baby died of SIDS, describes how you probably won't progress neatly through the "stages of grief." The long-term process of grief is better described as "two steps forward and one step back" (Whelan 2000).

Below are some reactions that many mothers, fathers, and other family members experience.

Overwhelming Sorrow

Especially in the initial days and weeks after you lose your baby, you may feel overwhelmed by sorrow. Your loss may hurt so much that you wonder if you are losing your mind. Some mothers feel that they are being swallowed by grief, and that they will never recover. Even when it stops being an almost constant presence, sorrow can come again in waves that sweep over you.

This deep sadness can also affect how you go about your day-to-day life. You may have trouble eating and sleeping, or find yourself seriously considering suicide. Even if you are not actively planning to take your own life, you may fantasize about going to sleep and not waking up, or about getting sick and dying so you can be with your baby.

Some mothers describe clinging to reminders of their babies, such as a favorite toy or a photograph, or continuing to wear maternity clothes. In your sorrow, your mind might start to play tricks on you. You might "hear" the baby crying or expect to see him lying in his crib. Your arms might ache to hold her and your breasts may fill with milk. You grieve with your whole body.

Numbness and Denial

Numbness and denial are two other common reactions. In the initial days and weeks after your baby dies, you may feel like you are in a fog, or that you are floating, watching this happen to someone else. You may not be able to even cry. It may feel like a dream from which you'll soon wake up and find your baby back with you.

Numbness and denial do serve a useful purpose. They temporarily shield you from pain and give you time to contemplate the unthinkable. Unfortunately, this reaction may also send the wrong message to people around you. Those closest to you may interpret your lack of tears or another strong reaction as an indication that you are "handling it well." When then numbness wears off in a few days or weeks, these same people may be surprised by your reaction and view this sudden display of emotion as "backtracking." Or the people who have gathered to support you may have gone home and back to their normal lives, leaving you alone to deal with your strongest feelings.

A Feeling of Unreality

In the days and weeks following the death of your baby, you may have a sense of unreality. You may feel surprised that life continues as before when you have been forever changed. This sense of unreality may be especially troubling if no one knew you were pregnant, or if your baby never left the hospital. You may have bonded with the hospital personnel, who knew your baby. But once your baby has died, you don't see the hospital personnel anymore. They now have other families to care for.

When you go back to your normal life, you are a different person. People in your life who want to spare you from pain may avoid talking about your baby. But you are in pain anyway, and not being able to talk about your baby just reinforces the unreality of the situation.

Others in your life may remove any trace of your baby before you even return from the hospital. Unfortunately, this may compound the problem for you. You may have wanted to smell the scent of your baby one more time in his clothes, or sit in the rocker where you planned to hold him. These things may be the only tangible connections you have with your baby. Even if you never brought your baby home, making your own decisions about the baby's things can help make this loss real to you, giving you an opportunity to say good-bye in your own time.

Anger and Rage

Anger can be one of the most persistent feelings you have. In the weeks, months, and even years following your baby's death, you may find that you are really, *really* angry. You may be mad that your partner did so little to support you when you needed him, or at his apparent lack of grief. You may be mad at things he said or did, or that he couldn't prevent the loss of your baby. Or your grief may be manifesting itself as anger, and your partner is simply a convenient target.

You may also find that you are mad at your mother, father, and siblings, or at other children you have. The stress of losing a child may bring other issues to the surface. Why are the other children all so healthy when your baby is gone? Why do they seem to need you so much? Why are they acting up now?

You may be mad at God. He could have protected your baby; why didn't he? You may wonder why this happened to you, especially when you've always tried to be a good person. Why would God take a baby that you really wanted when He gives babies to people who abuse them? How could a God of love allow you to suffer so much?

You may have been treated badly by medical personnel. The police may have insensitively implied that you had something to do with your baby's death. The hospital may have been more interested in your insurance information than in the fact that your baby just died. Your doctor or others may have tried to comfort you by saying: "You can have another one" or "At least this baby died before you got attached." Comments like that may actually destroy relationships you had prior to the loss of your baby, but most people say such things out of ignorance. Their lack of experience and discomfort with strong emotions can manifest itself in ways that are hurtful to you.

While anger may feel energizing and positive after being overwhelmed by grief, you must still be careful to express it in safe ways. Your anger is understandable and legitimate. But you can permanently damage your relationships with your partner, friends, family, or surviving children by lashing out at them. Deidre had a twin sister who died shortly after birth. One day, in a fit of anger, Deidre's mother told her that she wished that Terry had been the one who survived. Deidre has carried the pain of those angry words for many years, and it has created a rift between her and her mother.

Saul Bloom, whose son died of SIDS, suggests that you seek some form of physical release that will not harm you or others. He sought his by splitting wood and replacing plantings in his yard

(Whelan 2000). On those days when you feel overwhelmed by grief and anger, you might find that it helps to take a vigorous walk, throw rocks in your backyard, or hit a pillow. Writing in a journal or sharing with a support group can also be safe ways to vent your anger.

Isolation

Mothers who experience childbearing loss often find that they are left alone to grieve much of the time. People might avoid you because they don't know what to say. They may have children the same age that your child would have been, or they might be obviously pregnant or have a new baby, and worry that seeing their children may make you sad. They might even be afraid to associate too closely with someone whose baby has died because they fear it might happen to them.

You may find that the people in your life are supportive—to a point. At some time in the future, friends and family will expect you to get on with your life, and may be surprised that you are still grieving.

Finally, you may find that you cannot talk with other mothers who haven't lost children. Hearing them complain about their busyness makes you wish you could have even one more day of that kind of life. How can these women complain when they still have their precious children with them?

Guilt

Another very common reaction is guilt. Many mothers feel a profound sense of guilt, and wonder if they shouldn't have been able to "do something" that would have prevented their babies' death. Did activities during pregnancy contribute to your miscarriage or premature birth? Could your ambivalent feelings about being pregnant somehow have caused this to happen? You may have had an abortion earlier in your life, and with the loss of this baby, you are grieving for both.

You might feel guilty that you "let your child sleep," never dreaming that she was dead in her crib. If only you had checked on her sooner! Thinking back, you might remember every harsh word or thought. You remember the times when you finished what you were doing before going to get him, or the times when you were distracted, exhausted, and not enjoying every minute of time with your baby. If you had only known, you would have let the housework wait.

As you begin to work through your grief, you will start to have some good days. You may laugh occasionally and have times when you feel lighthearted. You'll have times when you enjoy the feeling of sun on your face, or the company of your partner, your children, or your friends. And then the guilty thought comes: If I'm enjoying myself, does that mean I don't care about my baby?

Depending on the circumstances surrounding your baby's death, you may feel guilty or regretful about other things that happened at the hospital. You may wish you had been there when your baby was removed from life support or died. You may wish that you had held him just one last time, taken pictures, saved a lock of her hair, or had a chance to say goodbye.

Mothers may be called upon to make decisions about how much intervention they wanted for their babies. These decisions are typically made for people at the end of life, rather than the beginning. Should my baby be placed on a ventilator or life support? Is this causing my baby pain? Should I just let her go? If you decided to take your baby off of life support, you may feel responsible for her death. If you decided to keep your baby on life support, you may feel responsible for the pain that he suffered.

Fear

If you have other children who are still living, you may find that you are fearful for them as well. You may stand and watch them for hours as they sleep to make sure that they are breathing. If you have subsequent children, you may be fearful through the entire pregnancy, and even until they are past the age when your first child died. Each childhood illness can cause you to hold your breath in apprehension. Once you've become personally aware of the fragility of life, you know that any moment you can lose someone else you love, as Kathy Whelan (2000) describes:

> Struck by tragedy once, I live waiting for the other shoe to drop. The first time Anna had a cold, I curled up in a fetal position, sure she would be dead by morning. The first time we took Michelle to the hospital for stomach pain, I was sure it was cancer. Every time Steve travels for business, I worry he will never return. I am emotionally tender. Unlike bones, which become stronger when broken, the heart gets weaker, the muscle tender. (191–192)

It may be years until you can approach others in a less fearful way.

Powerlessness

Powerlessness is another common reaction. You may have known that you were miscarrying, and realized that there was nothing you could do. Similarly, there was nothing you could do to keep your baby from dying. Sometimes you will assume guilt that is not yours because it is a way to counter powerlessness. Although guilt feels bad, it may seem preferable to the feeling that things were completely beyond your control.

Powerlessness is often compounded by events that occur during or after the death of your baby. Hospital routines can be overwhelming. You may have had an emergency cesarean, under general anesthetic. There may have been no time for the doctor and nurse attending you to even explain what was happening, or you may perceive that they were incompetent and allowed your baby to die.

After your baby's death, you may have been swept into the world of law enforcement. There may be an autopsy to determine the cause of death. You may even have been questioned as a suspect.

Loss of Identity

When a child dies, part of your identity gets lost too. If your first baby miscarried or died, are you still a mother? You may have had a miscarriage before you told anyone that you were pregnant. Do you tell people now that you had a miscarriage? On the other hand, can you carry on as if nothing has happened when part of you longs to scream, "My baby died!"?

Even when mothers have other children at home, or have children after one dies, there is often an awkwardness about what to tell people when they ask how many children you have. Do you acknowledge the child who died? You may not want to tell strangers that you lost a child. But to not acknowledge this child may make you feel deeply sad. Do you tell people that you have three children when you really have had four—or none when you have had one?

Depression

In the weeks and months following your baby's death, you may find that you are quite depressed, and are having trouble eating, sleeping, or even getting through the day. You might contemplate suicide. If you are depressed, it is important for you to get help soon. Don't try to go it alone. You might need a support group, one-on-one support from a counselor experienced in grief work, or both. You might also consider taking antidepressants until you feel like you can function again.

Your Other Children

Childbearing loss does not exist in a vacuum. It can affect how you feel about children you already have and those you have after your loss.

Children You Already Have

The loss of one child may make you fearful for your other children as well. You may find yourself being overprotective of them. You may also have days when you are overwhelmed by caring for them. They may provide a glimpse of life the way it used to be, or a sad reminder of what you have lost. Well-meaning friends and relatives might not know how to help you: Is it better to try to keep your other children away from you, or allow them to be near?

In the midst of your own grief, it can be hard to think about the needs of others. But your other children are grieving too, though they may express it in ways that seem inappropriate. Or they may be too young to fully understand why everyone seems so sad, and why their brother or sister is never coming home. They may sense the tension in the air and begin to act up, or they may be feeling guilty. Perhaps they had wished that the baby had never come to your family, and now feel responsible for his death. Your living children need to be able to express these kinds of concerns. While it is understandable that you might not feel up to meeting their dependency needs, recognize this and get some help. Bring in other caring adults so that your other children have one-on-one time to help them cope.

Should You Have Another Child?

This, of course, is a very personal decision. Some parents are too fearful to contemplate conceiving again quickly—or ever. You may decide not to have any more children. If you do make that decision, try not to take any permanent steps while you are in the midst of your grief. After grief recedes, you may find that you very much regret it.

Conversely, you might decide to get pregnant very soon after your baby dies. Your body may ache to hold another child. But it may be better to wait until the grief is not so raw before trying to get pregnant again. Consider also whether you are physically ready to conceive again. Your body may not have sufficiently recovered from your previous pregnancy.

It is also important that you realize that any subsequent child will never "replace" the child you lost. Your new baby will be his or her own person, and you cannot expect this new child to be just like your child who died. That is a heavy burden for a child to bear, and in the long run, it is not really fair for either of you.

Loss of a Multiple

Twins and higher-order multiples (triplets and more) are at increased risk for dying. One of your babies may have been weaker or smaller than the other(s) and did not survive. The baby may have died in utero, or after a stay in the NICU. You may find yourself in the unusual position of grieving while also caring for your surviving babies, as Tammy (2000) did:

> Everyone just expected me to be happy that I had a survivor. And I was, and I still am. I endured (and am still enduring) both joy and grief in one. I am thrilled to have Matthew and have him doing well, but I am incredibly saddened that I don't have Mark. Everyone around me expected me to just go on and not truly grieve for Mark. Even family members.

See the resource list at the end of this chapter for Web sites that address the loss of a multiple.

There are also physical challenges associated with loss of a multiple. You may have one or more preemies to mother at home, while needing to also be at the NICU. It should come as no surprise that you spend your first few weeks or months in a state of perpetual exhaustion.

What You Can Do

There is nothing you can do that will bring your baby back. But there are steps you can take that will help you heal, and bring some closure to your experience.

Take Care of Yourself Physically

In the aftermath of any significant loss, your body becomes more vulnerable to illness. As I described in chapter 2, a flood of stress hormones suppresses the immune system. Unfortunately, in the wake of a baby's death, you may find that you cannot sleep or eat, and that you are up most of the day taking care of other people's needs. Suddenly, you become quite ill too. Even though you don't feel like doing it, it is important that you take care of your health. Physical self-care is an important part of your grief work.

You might also consider incorporating regular massage into your self-care regimen. We often carry severe grief in our bodies as well as our hearts and minds. Massage will help dissipate some of the stress your body carries and will also boost your immune system.

Take Care of Yourself Emotionally

You also need help and support as you grieve. Finding support may be harder than it first appears. Family members may be supportive at first, but then expect you to get on with your life.

The stress of a baby's death may put a significant strain on your relationship with your partner. Your partner may be grieving in a very different way than you. Men and women have very different culturally sanctioned ways of dealing with feelings. For example, you may need to talk about what happened as a way to process your feelings and make what happened seem more real. Your partner may find that talking about it makes him feel worse, and that for him, the most effective strategy is just not to think about it. It is easy to fall into a situation where each partner feels that the other is being insensitive to his or her needs. Each family member needs permission to grieve in his or her own way.

That being said, you need to give yourself permission to seek support outside of your family or your relationship with your partner, if you cannot get what you need inside your family. A support group for parents who have experienced similar losses may be lifesaving for you, as can a therapist who specializes in grief work.

Don't forget the Internet as a possible source of support and healing. There are many sites dedicated to all types of infant loss. Even if you choose not to share your story online, you may find it helpful to read about the experiences of others. This support is available twenty-four hours a day—a boon if you are having trouble sleeping.

Finally, although this is not technically "support," you might find it helpful to write about your experiences. Writing offers you a safe place to vent some of your feelings, and can help you understand and gain perspective on your experience. If you have never journaled before, you might want to check out *Opening Up* by James Pennebaker (1997). This book describes research demonstrating the psychological and emotional benefits of processing difficult experiences in writing, and gives specific suggestions for getting the most benefit out of this activity.

Find a Way to Memorialize Your Baby

One of the difficulties of pregnancy loss or infant death is that there is little left to memorialize your baby's life. The experience will seem more real to you if you can find a concrete way to remember your baby. If you haven't done so already, you might consider holding a memorial service. Some people remember their babies by planting a tree, making a donation, or setting up a charitable fund. Even putting together a scrapbook or photo album can mark your baby's time with you, however brief. One of my neighbors lost a little girl at the age of four. Every year, she puts up a Christmas tree with only angel ornaments on it to commemorate her daughter.

Work toward Acceptance

Be realistic about how much recovery you expect. You can adapt to what has happened, but it is not something you "get over" or forget. Your experience has most likely changed the way you look at the world, and you will never be the person you were before. But you can learn to live again, experience joy again, and love other children. Many women have turned their personal sorrows into strengths, and have used their experiences to reach out to others. Ten years after the death of her baby to SIDS, Kathy Whelan (2000) describes her journey toward healing this way:

> The hardest part of survival is acceptance. Accepting who I am, a mother who has lost a son. Accepting that Mikey was here, and that I lost him. I can no longer mother Mikey, but I can mother other people who have had similar losses.
>
> And so, almost 10 years after losing my son, I am surviving. No, I am thriving. I faced the fears of having children again. I lived through five pregnancies, one mis-

carriage, and three first years of worry. I am raising three beautiful children. They are loving, affectionate, creative. I have used my pain to write meaningful stories and poems that have touched other people's hearts. I have used my creativity as an outlet for the love of my dead son, a son who may never see my work, but who lives in my heart because of my work. I have been an example of survival to other parents who are just beginning their grief journeys. I have used my pain to show my children the depths of my love for them.

I love how my Dad explained grief. With time, grief would find a place in my heart where it could live peacefully. And every now and then, I could take out my grief and feel its overpowering sadness. The feelings would be similar to those I first felt, but they would not take control of my every waking thought. And so I bear my grief for Mikey in my heart, close to the surface of my soul. And every once in a while, my grief, my love pours out, reminding me of the passion I had for my first-born son. And I can live with that. (192)

Surviving the death of your baby will probably be the hardest thing you ever do. But as the mothers who have shared their stories in this chapter will tell you, there is hope. You can go on. In closing, I'd like to share the words of Linda DeYmaz, from her remarkably touching book *Mommy, Please Don't Cry* (1996):

> Someday, Mommy, we will hold each other tight!
> Then you will cradle me in you arms,
> And stroke my hair . . .
> And once again, our hearts will beat
> together.
>
> Mommy, please don't cry . . .
> I'll wait right here for you.

For Further Reading

There are some excellent resources available to mothers and fathers who have experienced childbearing losses. You'll have times when you want to read everything you can find, and others when you don't want to read anything at all. Give yourself permission to grieve at your own pace and in your own way. There is also a lot of information available on the Internet. If you are not the type of person who likes support groups, or you do not live in a place where there is one nearby, these sites may be a lifeline to you.

Resources for All Types of Infant Loss

These books and Web sites describe all types of infant loss. All are good. You may find them especially helpful if you have experienced more than one type of loss. Davis, O'Keefe Lafser, and Panuthos and Romeo's books are especially good resources for miscarriage and infertility.

Davis, D. L. 1996. *Empty Cradle, Broken Heart: Surviving the Death of Your Baby.* Golden, Colo.: Fulcrum Publishing.

O'Keefe Lafser, C. 1998. *An Empty Cradle: A Full Heart. Reflections for Mothers and Fathers after Miscarriage, Stillbirth, or Infant Death.* Chicago: Loyola.

Panuthos, C., and C. Romeo. 1984. *Ended Beginnings: Healing Childbearing Losses.* Westport, Conn.: Bergin and Garvey.

Center for Loss in Multiple Births (CLIMB): www.climb-support.org

Multiple Angels Network: www.angels4ever.com

Parents of Multiples Forever: www.erichad.com

A Place to Remember: www.aplacetoremember.com

Resources for Sudden Infant Death Syndrome

Sears, W. 1995. *SIDS: A Parent's Guide to Understanding and Preventing Sudden Infant Death Syndrome.* New York: Little, Brown.

Whelan, K. A. 2000. *Grief Songs: Stories, Letters, and Poems That Chronicle the Recovery and Survival of a Community after the Sudden Death of a Baby.* Boston: Massachusetts Center for Sudden Infant Death Syndrome. Available from the Massachusetts Center for SIDS, Boston Medical Center, One Boston Medical Center Place, Boston, MA 02118; 800-641-7437.

National SIDS Resource Center: www.circsol.com/SIDS

SIDS Alliance: www.sidsalliance.org

SIDS Network: ww.sids-network.org

Resources for Miscarriage and Infertility

Diamond, K. 1991. *Motherhood after Miscarriage.* Holbrook, Mass.: Adams Media.

Hygeia Foundation: www.hygeia.org

InterNational Council on Infertility Information Dissemination: www.inciid.org

IVF.com: www.ivf.com

Resolve: www.resolve.org

Women's Health Information: Search for "recurrent miscarriage" at www.womens-health.co.uk

A Book That Shares Mothers' Stories

Sometimes, the most helpful thing you can do is read the stories of others who have experienced similar losses. Many of the Websites that I have listed also share stories, as do Christine O'Keeffe Lafser and Kathy Whelan's books listed earlier.

DeYmaz, L. 1996. *Mommy, Please Don't Cry.* Sisters, Ore.: Multnomah Publishers. This amazing little book deserves some special comment. It looks like a children's book, but is written for mothers from the baby's perspective. Many mothers have been touched by this book. It is written from an explicitly Christian point of view.

Epilogue

In the introduction to this book, I encouraged you to think about making positive changes in your life. But you may not know where to begin. In these last pages, I want to bring some of the threads together and help you find a starting place.

Identify the Positives in Your Life

Throughout this book, I've described the difficulties you face as a mother. To help you identify problem areas, I needed to focus on the negatives. Now I want you to refocus. Take a minute and think about what is going well.

I learned this principle from two unlikely sources. The first was Julie Morgenstern's *Organizing from the Inside Out* (1998). Julie is a professional organizer. The very definition of her job is to help people recognize problem areas in their lives. Yet she states that when you are looking to make a change, you should first consider what is working for you now. That way, you build changes on strengths you already have.

Jon Kabat-Zinn, in *Full Catastrophe Living* (1991), teaches the same principle. Jon teaches mindfulness meditation to patients at University of Massachusetts Medical Center. Many of his patients are critically, or even terminally, ill. Yet he encourages them to see that no matter how sick they are, more is right with their bodies than wrong. I first read this at a time when I was very ill, and it really struck me. When you are sick, there is a tendency to focus on what's not working. He provided the broader picture, and made me see beyond my immediate health crisis.

You can apply the same principle. Right now, you may feel overwhelmed by your life. You may see only problems. But if you can identify even one strength, you can start by building on that.

Take Time Out for Self-Care

This is also a good time to start treating your body right. You may think that you have "no time" to exercise, eat well, and relax. But think of it this way: if you had a total breakdown of your health, somehow your work would still be there. Mothering is a marathon, not a sprint. If you are going to be there for the long haul, you must start investing in your future health now.

Change Your Daily Work

Start paying attention to your daily tasks: those you like, and those you don't. Focus on the tasks you dislike. Can you change them? For example, if you're employed and your job is the source of stress, think about how to make it better. Can you change jobs? Can you reduce your hours or work out a more flexible arrangement? Can you take some classes to increase your skills? Elaine St. James, in *Living the Simple Life* (1999), has lots of practical suggestions on how you can change your daily work. You may not be able to make changes now, but you can make a plan. Knowing that you have a way out, even if it is several years down the road, can help make the present situation more tolerable. By identifying particular trouble spots, you can start to think of solutions, rather than writing off your whole situation as impossible.

Start Laughing Again

I talk with mothers all the time, and can't help but notice that we can be a grim bunch. We take ourselves much too seriously. King Solomon said that "a merry heart does good like medicine" (Proverbs 17:22). Science is finally confirming what he knew. Laughing and a lightness of spirit enhances the immune system and makes us feel better. But when we are stressed, our sense of humor often vanishes.

If you are out of practice, here are some suggestions to revive your sense of humor. Rent or borrow some funny movies. Read some funny books. Keep a stash of humorous materials on hand and pull them out whenever stress starts getting the better of you. Also, learn to appreciate the natural joy of children. Many things that happen in our everyday lives are quite comical. We have to stop being so intense, and learn to see the joy and humor around us.

Seek a Mothering Mentor

When we are in the midst of our own daily struggles, it is easy to lose sight of the big picture. You may wonder if what you are slaving for each day makes any difference. A mothering mentor can be a tremendous source of encouragement. When you are in the midst of day-to-day child care, you may believe that this stage will last "forever." Talking with older women can help you realize how quickly this time goes when looked at from the perspective of a whole life. My one caution would be for you to seek the advice of women who had positive mothering experiences. Just because a woman is older, you cannot assume that she enjoyed her time as a mother. A mother who is bitter about her mothering experience can reinforce some of the negative feelings you are trying to eliminate. Someone can be honest about the difficulties and challenges of mothering, but still have an overall positive experience. Seek these women out.

Go Online

If you are not already connected to the Internet, I would encourage you to think about it. Throughout this book, I've given you information on Web sites relevant to specific issues. While there is a lot of garbage on the Internet, there is also an amazing amount of information and support available. As with anything, you must be a wise consumer, and be selective about what you read.

Many public libraries now have Internet access, if you can't afford a computer. University extension and other adult education programs regularly have classes to get you started. And don't forget your kids. Older kids can probably find their way around pretty well, and can show you how.

Learn to Pace Yourself

So often we wear ourselves out thinking that everything needs to be done *now*. We labor under the false belief that if we only work hard enough, we can do it all. Recognize that this is a lie. There will always be stuff to do, but it doesn't all have to be done today.

Besides, people who learn to take breaks and pace themselves are actually more productive.

Consider Hiring a Coach

If you want some assistance beyond what you can get in a book, you might consider hiring a personal coach. Personal coaches are not therapists, nor are they sports coaches. Rather, they help people make choices so that they are living by their own values. If you want more information, the Web site for Coach U is www.coachu.com. This is a referral service divided by state, country, or the issue you want to address.

Cultivate a Spiritual Life

Like many of you, I have specific religious beliefs and am not entirely comfortable recommending a generic "spirituality." On the other hand, I would be remiss if I did not mention the amazing health benefits of faith, prayer, and meditation. People with religious beliefs typically live longer and have better health and stronger relationships than people who don't. My colleagues in psychology are somewhat baffled by these findings, and don't know what to do with them. But even they can see that a spiritual life makes a difference (Benson 1997).

Surround Yourself with Beauty

My final suggestion has to do with nourishing your soul. Do this for yourself and your family. When we're stressed, we tend to be utilitarian. Or labor under the mistaken belief that beauty is for the rich alone. We think of great works of art, or lovely pieces of furniture rather than realizing that beauty is something we can unearth even in our own homes. Fortunately, beauty is something that we all can have for very little cost.

Sometimes, you can dramatically increase the levels of beauty around you with things you already have. Can you group items more attractively? Can you bring out some family heirlooms or other things you love? Can you attractively frame some of your photographs? Can you bring more color to a room? Reducing clutter can dramatically improve the looks of a room. Look around your home. Do you love the stuff that is there? If not, why are you keeping it? If you can't improve it, consider moving it to another location, selling it, or giving it away. Learn to make conscious choices about what you have around you.

Beauty is not limited to our sense of sight. Our sense of hearing can experience beauty too. Listen to good music. It doesn't have to be "classical," although there are some very good collections available. But it should be music that makes your spirit soar. Many public libraries have great collections of tapes and CDs you can borrow for free. Or perhaps you can swap with a friend. Fortunately, music is a very inexpensive source of beauty.

Think also of smell. It's great to have a home or workplace that smells good. Different scents can also improve your alertness (peppermint) or your mood (citrus), promote relaxation (lavender), or evoke images of a cozy home (baking bread, cinnamon). Try thinking about ways that you can incorporate nice smells into your everyday life.

Taste is another way that you can incorporate beauty. If you're not confident in the kitchen, learn some basic cooking techniques so you can eat good food. Often, simply prepared food is best. Glenna Matthews, in *"Just a Housewife"* (1987), describes the "dumbing down" of the American palate with the mass production of convenience foods. We've lost our taste for fresh vegetables, succulently prepared meats, and fresh fruits. As we create workspaces in our kitchens that are more pleasant, perhaps we can once again enjoy the delights of a home-cooked meal.

Finally, don't forget beauty that is experienced through our sense of touch. Do you have a comfortable place to sit in your home? Home furnishings can be pretty uncomfortable. Don't sacrifice comfort for looks. Also, be sure to have places where people can sit comfortably together. Many times, families don't have enough seating for everyone to be together at the same time. This small change can yield big dividends for your family.

And so we've come to the end of our journey together. Mothering is a tough job, but can be one of your proudest lifetime achievements. The work you are doing is vital to the next generation. In closing, I'd like to leave you with the thoughts of Alexandra Stoddard in her book *Mothers: A Celebration*:

> The word mother conjures up more than a person. A mother is a life force, a spirit. She is living, loving energy, channeling abundance into all of our lives. Being a mother is about having children, but her influence extends far beyond her own offspring. She is a universal person. Her

strength comes gently. What makes her strong is her inherent maternal instincts. A mother is the greatest force in the world.

All females are part of this universal generous energy. Collectively, women nourish, guide, and provide continuity.

Mothers mother. That's what we do. That's who we are. Bless you.

REFERENCES

Abramowitz, J. N., and A. T. Mattoon. 1999. *Cutting the Costs of Paper: Saving Forests, Water, Energy . . . and Money.* Worldwatch Institute, www.worldwatch.org.

Affluenza. 2000. www.pbs.org.

Alexander P., et al. 1998. Adult attachment and long-term effects in survivors of incest. *Child Abuse & Neglect* 22:45–61.

American Association for Premature Infants. 2000. www.aapi-online.org

American Debt Management Services. 1998. Debt and credit card statistics. www.beevy.com/american/statistics?58-2749.

Amundson, K. 2000. Breaking the cycle of violence. *Consortium Connections* 9:8.

Armey, D. 1996. Time is money: Economic crunch is taking time from parents and children. *World,* August 3/10, 24.

Ascione, F. R. 1995. *Domestic Violence and Cruelty to Animals.* Paper presented at the Fourth International Family Violence Research Conference, Durham, N.H., July.

Aslett, D. 1984. *Clutter's Last Stand.* Cincinnati: Writer's Digest Books.

———. 2000. *No Time to Clean.* Pocatello, Ida.: Marsh Creek Press.

Atkinson, H. 1985. *Women and Fatigue.* New York: Pocket Books.

Avissar, S., Y. Nechamkin, G. Roitman, and G. Schreiber. 1997. Reduced G protein functions and immunoreactive levels in mononuclear leukocytes of patients with depression. *American Journal of Psychiatry* 154:211–217.

Baker Miller, J. 1995. *Toward a New Psychology of Women.* Boston: Beacon Press.

Banyard, V. 1997. The impact of childhood sexual abuse and family functioning on four dimensions of women's later parenting. *Child Abuse & Neglect* 21:1095–1107.

Barrett, J. H., P. Brennan, M. Fiddler, and A. Silman. 2000. Breastfeeding and postpartum relapse in women with rheumatoid arthritis and inflammatory arthritis. *Arthritis & Rheumatism* 43:1010–1015.

Becker-Lausen, E., and S. Mallon-Kraft. 1997. Pandemic outcomes: The intimacy variable. In *Out of Darkness: Contemporary Perspectives on Family Violence,* edited by G. K. Kantor and J. Jasinski. Newbury Park, Calif.: Sage Publications.

Beecher Stowe, H. 1853, 1997. *Uncle Tom's Cabin.* New York: Dutton Signet.

Benson, H., with M. Stark. 1997. *Timeless Healing: The Power and Biology of Belief.* New York: Fireside.

Bifulco, A., T. Harris, and G. W. Brown. 1992. Mourning or early inadequate care? Reexamining the relationship of maternal loss in childhood with adult depression and anxiety. *Development & Psychopathology* 4:433–451.

Blumberg, N. L. 1980. Effects of neonatal risk, maternal attitude, and cognitive style on early postpartum adjustment. *Journal of Abnormal Psychology* 89:139–150.

Blumenthal, M. 1999. *The Complete German Commision E Monographs: Therapeutic Guide to Herbal Medicine.* Newton, Mass.: Integrative Medicine Communication.

Brabec, B. 1997. *Homemade Money: How to Select, Start, Manage, Market and Multiply the Profits of a Business at Home.* Cincinnati: F & W Publications.

Brady, D. 2000. Martha Inc.: Inside the growing empire of America's lifestyle queen. *Business Week Online,* www.businessweek.com, January, 17.

Brandt, A. 1998. *Understanding and Acknowledging Negative Emotions.* ElderCare Online, www.ec-online.net.

Breathnach, S. B. 1995. *Simple Abundance: A Daybook of Comfort and Joy.* New York: Warner Books.

Bremner, J. D., S. M. Southwick, D. R. Johnson, R. Yehuda, and D. S. Charney. 1993. Childhood physical abuse and combat-related posttraumatic stress disorder in Vietnam veterans. *American Journal of Psychiatry* 150:235–239.

Briere, J. N., and D. M. Elliot. 1994. Immediate and long-term impacts of child sexual abuse. *The Future of Children* 4:54–69.

Bryson, K., and L. M. Casper. 1998. Current populaation reports. *Household Characteristics March 1997.* Washington, D.C.: U.S. Department of Commerce.

Buck, P. S. 1941. *Of Men and Women.* New York: John Day.

Buist, A. 1998. Childhood abuse, postpartum depression and parenting difficulties: A literature review of associations. *Australian and New Zealand Journal of Psychiatry* 32:370–378.

Burkett, L. 1999. *Women Leaving the Workplace: How to Make the Transition from Work to Home.* Chicago: Moody Press.

Burns, D. 1989. *The Feeling Good Handbook.* New York: Penguin.

———. 1999. *Feeling Good: The New Mood Therapy.* New York: Avon.

Cain, N. 1996. *Healing the Child: A Mother's Story.* New York: Rawson Associates.

Cardozo, A. R. 1996. *Sequencing: A New Solution for Women Who Want Marriage, Career and Family.* San Bernardino, Calif.: Borgo Press.

Cassidy, A. 1999. Time squeeze: Can working moms beat the clock? Results from our exclusive survey. *Working Mother,* November, 48–54.

Cassidy, J., and P. R. Shaver. 1999. *Handbook of Attachment: Theory, Research, and Clinical Applications.* New York: Guilford.

Centers for Disease Control and Prevention. 1999. *National Vital Statistics Reports* 47. www.cdc.gov.

Cloud, H., and J. Townsend. 1992. *Boundaries: When to Say "Yes," When to Say "No." Take Control of Your Life.* Grand Rapids, Mich.: Zondervan.

Covey, S. R. 1989. *The Seven Habits of Highly Effective People.* New York: Fireside.

Crockenberg, S., and K. McCluskey. 1986. Change in maternal behavior during the baby's first year of life. *Child Development* 57:746–753.

Cutrona, C. E., and B. R. Troutman. 1986. Social support, infant temperament, and parenting self-efficacy: A mediational model of postpartum depression. *Child Development* 57:1507–1518.

Dacyczyn, A. 1992. *The Tightwad Gazette.* New York: Villard Books.

———. 1995. *The Tightwad Gazette II.* New York: Villard Books.

———. 1996. *The Tightwad Gazette III.* New York: Villard Books.

Davidson, J. 1991. *Breathing Space: Living and Working at a Comfortable Pace in a Sped-Up Society.* New York: MasterMedia.

Davis, D. L. 1996. *Empty Cradle, Broken Heart: Surviving the Death of Your Baby.* Golden, Colo.: Fulcrum Publishing.

DeYmaz, L. 1996. *Mommy, Please Don't Cry.* Sisters, Org.: Multnomah Press.

Diamond, K. 1991. *Motherhood after Miscarriage.* Holbrook, Mass.: Adams Media.

Dominguez, J., and V. Robin. 1992. *Your Money or Your Life: Transforming Your Relationship with Money and Achieving Financial Independence.* New York: Viking.

Earle, A. M. 1898, 1992. *Home Life in Colonial Days.* Stockbridge, Mass.: Berkshire House.

Egeland, B., D. Jacobvitz, and L. A. Sroufe. 1988. Breaking the cycle of abuse. *Child Development* 59:1080–1088.

Fidler, A. T., and J. Bernstein. 1999. Infertility: From a personal to a public health problem. *Public Health Reports* 114:494–511.

Finkelhor, D. 1994. Current information on the scope and nature of child sexual abuse. *Future of Children* 4:31–53.

Fisher, D. G. 1996. Mothers at home. *New Beginnings,* September/October, 132–135.

Friedan, B. 1963. *The Feminine Mystique.* New York: Dell.

Fuller, J. A., and R. Warner. 2000. Family stressors as predictors of codependency. *Genetic, Social, and General Psychology Monographs* 126:5–22.

Gara, M. A., L. A. Allen, E. P. Herzog, and R. L. Woolfolk. 2000. The abused child as parent: The structure and content of physically abused mothers' perceptions of their babies. *Child Abuse & Neglect* 24:627–639.

Gibson, R. L., and T. S. Hartshorne. 1996. Childhood sexual abuse and adult loneliness and network orientation. *Child Abuse & Neglect* 20:1087–1093.

Goldberg, B. 1998. *Alternative Medicine Guide to Chronic Fatigue, Fibromyalgia, and Environmental Illness: 26 Doctors Show You How They Reverse These Con-*

ditions with Clinically Proven Alternative Therapies. Tiburon, Calif.: Future Medicine Press.

Greenspan, M. 1998. "Exceptional" mothering in a "normal" world. In *Mothering Against the Odds: Diverse Voices of Contemporary Mothers,* edited by C. Garcia Coll, J. L. Surrey, and K. Weingarten. New York: Guilford.

Gromada, K. 1999. *Mothering Multiples.* Schaumburg, Ill.: La Leche League International.

Hale, T. W. 1999. *Medications and Mothers' Milk.* Amarillo, Tex.: Pharmasoft Medical Publishing.

Hammonds, K. H. 1998. There really aren't enough hours in the day. *Business Week Online,* www.businessweek.com, April 15.

Health. 2000. The alarming truth about his snoring. *Health,* January/February, 22.

Hochschild, A., with A. Machung. 1989. *The Second Shift.* New York: Avon Books.

Hochschild, A. R. 1997. *The Time Bind: When Work Becomes Home and Home Becomes Work.* New York: Metropolitan Books.

Holden, C. 2000. Global survey examines impact of depression. *Science* 288:39–40.

Hunfeld, J. A., A. Tempels, J. Passchier, and F. W. J. Hazebroek. 1999. Parental burden and grief one year after the birth of a child with a congenital anomaly. *Journal of Pediatric Psychology* 24:515–520.

Isenberg, D. A. 1999. *Complicated Systemic Lupus Erythematous: How to Assess It, How to Treat It.* Address at the annual meetings of American College of Rheumatology, Boston, Mass., November.

Jarvis, P. A., B. J. Myers, and G. L. Creasey. 1989. The effects of infants' illness on mothers' interactions with prematures at 4 and 8 months. *Infant Behavior and Development* 12:25–35.

Johnson, J. G., P. Cohen, J. Brown, E. M. Smailes, and D. P. Bernstein. 1999. Childhood maltreatment increases risk for personality disorders during early adulthood. *Archives of General Psychiatry* 56:600–606.

Johnson, S. K. 2000. Chore wars. *Ladies' Home Journal,* March.

Kabat-Zinn, J. 1991. *Full Catastrophe Living: Using the Wisdom of Your Body and Mind to Face Stress, Pain and Illness.* New York: Dell Publishing Company.

Kelch, S. 1999. Another option for fighting the blues. *Herbs for Health,* September/October, 74–75.

Kendall-Tackett, K. A. 2000. Physiological correlates of childhood abuse: Chronic hyperarousal in PTSD, depression and irritable bowel syndrome. *Child Abuse & Neglect* 24:799–810.

Kendall-Tackett, K. A., with G. Kaufman Kantor. 1993. *Postpartum Depression: A Comprehensive Approach for Nurses.* Newbury Park, Calif.: Sage Publications.

Kendall-Tackett, K. A., and R. Marshall. 1999. Victimization and diabetes: An exploratory study. *Child Abuse & Neglect* 23:593–596.

Kendall-Tackett, K. A., R. Marshall, and K. E. Ness. 2000. Victimization, healthcare use, and health maintenance. *Family Violence & Sexual Assault Bulletin* 16:18–21.

Kendall-Tackett, K. A., L. M. Williams, and D. Finkelhor. 1993. The impact of sexual abuse on children: A review and synthesis of recent empirical studies. *Psychological Bulletin* 113:164–180.

Khalsa, K. P. S. 2000. Don't take your herbs for granted. *Herbs for Health*, July/August, 52–55.

Kiely, J. L., J. C. Kleinman, and M. Kiely. 1992. Triplets and higher-order multiple births: Time trends and infant mortality. *American Journal of Diseases of Childhood* 146:862–868.

Kitzinger, S. 1990. *The Crying Baby*. New York: Penguin.

Koocher, G. 2000. Personal communication with author.

Koverola, C., and M. Morahan. 2000. *Differential Impact of Exposure to Domestic Violence and Child Sexual Abuse: Maternal Functioning as a Meditating Variable*. Paper presented at "Victimization of Children and Youth: An International Research Conference." Durham, N.H., July.

Kurcinka, M. S. 1991. *Raising Your Spirited Child: A Guide for Parents Whose Child Is More*. New York: HarperPerennial.

LaPlante, M. P., D. Carlson, H. S. Kaye, and J. E. Bradsher. 1996. *Families with Diabilities in the United States: Executive Summary*. Washington, D.C.: U.S. Department of Health and Human Services.

Leman, K. 1987. *Women Who Try Too Hard: Breaking the Pleaser Habits*. Grand Rapids, Mich.: Fleming H. Revell.

Lemieux, A. M., and C. L. Coe. 1995. Abuse-related post-traumatic stress disorder: Evidence for chronic neuroendocrine activation in women. *Psychosomatic Medicine* 57:105–115.

Lenz, E., and A. Baugh-Meyer. 2000. The scary herbs: Are they really so scary? *Herbs for Health*, July/August, 48–51.

Lewis, D. S., with G. Lewis. 1989. *Motherhood Stress*. Dallas, Tex.: Word Publishing.

M. C. 1893, 1995. *Everybody's Book of Correct Conduct, Being the Etiquette of Every-day Life*. London: Saxon and Co.

Mack, D. 1997. *The Assault on Parenthood: How Our Culture Undermines the Family*. New York: Simon and Schuster.

Marco, C. A., J. E. Schwartz, J. M. Neale, S. Shiffman, D. Catley, and A. Stone. 2000. Impact of gender and having children in the household on ambulatory blood pressure in work and nonwork settings: A partial replication and new findings. *Annals of Behavioral Medicine* 22:110–115.

Matthews, G. 1987. *"Just a Housewife": The Rise and Fall of Domesticity in America*. New York: Oxford University Press.

McCormick, L. 1995. Depression in mothers of children with Attention Deficit Hyperactivity Disorder. *Family Medicine* 27:176–179.

McGrath, E., G. P. Keita, B. R. Strickland, and N. F. Russo. 1990. *Women and Depression: Risk Factors and Treatment Issues*. Washington, D.C.: American Psychological Association.

McGuire, P. A. 1999. Worker stress, health reaching critical point. *APA Monitor Online*, www.apa.org/monitor, May.

McMillen, C., S. Zuravin, and G. Rideout. 1995. Perceived benefit from child sexual abuse. *Journal of Consulting and Clinical Psychology* 63:1037–1043.

Mintz, S., and S. Kellogg. 1988. *Domestic Revolutions: A Social History of American Family Life.* New York: Free Press.

Moran, V. 1997. *Shelter for the Spirit: Create Your Own Haven in a Hectic World.* New York: HarperPerennial.

———. 1999. *Creating a Charmed Life: Sensible, Spiritual Secrets Every Busy Woman Should Know.* New York: HarperSanFrancisco.

Morgenstern, J. 1998. *Organizing from the Inside Out.* New York: Henry Holt and Company.

Murray, B. 2000. Family income predicts children's postdivorce well-being. *Monitor on Psychology,* June, 14.

Murray, M. T. 1996. *Natural Alternatives to Prozac.* New York: William Morrow & Co.

Myers, N. 2000. Sustainable consumption. *Science* 287:2419.

National Academy on an Aging Society. 2000. *Caregiving: Helping the Elderly with Activity Limitations,* www.agingsociety.org.

National Institute of Child Health and Human Development. 1999. Chronicity of maternal depressive symptoms, maternal sensitivity, and child functioning at 36 months. *Developmental Psychology* 35:1297-1310.

National Institute of Mental Health. 2000a. *NIMH Research on Treatment for Attention Deficit Hyperactivity Disorder (ADHD): The Multimodal Treatment Study.* www.nimh.nih.gov.

National Institute of Mental Health. 2000b. *Attention Deficit Hyperactivity Disorder.* www.nimh.nih.gov.

National Sleep Foundation. 2000a. *2000 Omnibus Sleep in America Poll.* www.sleepfoundation.org.

———. 2000b. *The Nature of Sleep.* www.sleepfoundation.org.

Nelson, M. E., with S. Wernick. 1998. *Strong Women Stay Young.* New York: Bantam.

Olkin, R. 1999. *What Psychotherapists Should Know about Disability.* New York: Guilford.

O'Neil, J. R. 1993. *The Paradox of Success: When Winning at Work Means Losing at Life.* New York: G. P. Putnam's Sons.

Panuthos, C., and C. Romeo. 1984. *Ended Beginnings: Healing Childbearing Losses.* Westport, Conn.: Bergin & Garvey.

Pennebaker, J. W. 1997. *Opening Up: The Healing Power of Expressing Emotions.* New York: Guilford.

Polansky, N. A., J. M. Gaudin, P. W. Ammons, and K. B. Davis. 1985. The psychological ecology of the neglectful mother. *Child Abuse & Neglect* 9:265–275.

Potter, B. 1998. *Overcoming Job Burnout: How to Renew Enthusiasm for Work.* Berkeley, Calif.: Ronin.

Preston, J., and J. Johnson. 1997. *Clinical Psychopharmacology Made Ridiculously Simple.* 3rd ed. Miami: MedMaster, Inc.

Radke-Yarrow, M. 1998. *Children of Depressed Mothers.* Cambridge, U.K.: Cambridge University Press.

Raskin, V. 1997. *When Words Are Not Enough: The Women's Prescription for Depression and Anxiety.* New York: Broadway.

Rhoades, N., and S. Hutchinson. 1994. Labor experiences of child sexual abuse survivors. *Birth* 21:213–220.

Robins, V. 1994. *A Declaration of Independence from Overconsumption.* New Road Map Foundation, www.newroadmap.org.

Rosenthal, N. E. 1998. *Winter Blues: Seasonal Affective Disorder. What it Is and How to Overcome It.* New York: Guilford.

St. James, E. 1999. *Living the Simple Live: A Guide to Scaling Down and Enjoying More.* New York: Hyperion.

Sapolsky, R. M. 1996. Why stress is bad for your brain. *Science* 273:749–750.

Schor, J. 1992. *The Overworked American: The Unexpected Decline of Leisure.* New York: Basic Books.

Schwartz, F. N., with J. Zimmerman. 1992. *Breaking with Tradition: Women and Work, the New Facts of Life.* New York: Warner Books.

Schwartz Cowan, R. 1983. *More Work for Mother: The Ironies of Household Technology from the Open Hearth to the Microwave.* New York: Basic Books.

Scoon-Rogers, L. 1999. *Child Support for Custodial Mothers and Fathers: 1995.* Washington, D.C.: U.S. Department of Commerce, Economics and Statistics Administration. www.census.gov.

Sears, W. 1991. *Christian Parenting and Childcare.* Nashville, Tenn.: Thomas Nelson.

———. 1995. *SIDS: A Parent's Guide to Understanding and Preventing Sudden Infant Death Syndrome.* New York: Little, Brown.

Sears, W., and M. Sears. 1996. *Parenting the Fussy Baby and High-Need Child.* New York: Little, Brown.

Sears, W., and L. Thompson. 1998. *The A.D.D. Book: New Understandings, New Approaches to Parenting Your Child.* New York: Little, Brown.

Sedlak, A., and D. D. Broadhurst. 1996. *Third National Incidence Study of Child Abuse and Neglect,* Final Report. Washington, D.C.: U.S. Department of Health and Human Services.

Smith, B., J. L. Surrey, and M. Watkins. 1998. "Real mothers": Adoptive mothers resisting marginization and re-creating motherhood. In *Mothering Against the Odds: Diverse Voices of Contemporary Mothers,* edited by C. Garcia Coll, J. L. Surrey, and K. Weingarten. New York: Guilford.

Solomon, Z., and K. Ginsburg. 1999. Aging in the shadow of war. In *Post-Traumatic Stress Disorder: A Lifespan Development Perspective,* edited by A. Maerchkern, M. Schutzwohltz, and Z. Solomon. Seattle: Hognefe and Huber Publishers.

Stan, A. 2000. Woman on the verge: On the eve of her run for the Senate, Hillary Rodham Clinton reflects on a very public life in transition. *Working Woman,* September, 60–63.

Stoddard, A. 1988. *Living a Beautiful Life: 500 Ways to Add Elegance, Order, Beauty and Joy to Every Day of Your Life.* New York: Morrow.

———. 1992. *Creating a Beautiful Home.* New York: Avon Books.

———. 1996. *Gracious Living in the New World: Finding Joy in Changing Times.* New York: Avon Books.

———. 1996. *Mothers: A Celebration.* New York: Avon.

Sullivan, P. M., and J. F. Knutson. 2000. Maltreatment and disabilities: A population-based epidemiological study. *Child Abuse & Neglect* 24:1257–1273.

Swindle, R., K. Heller, B. Pescosolido, and S. Kikuzawa. 2000. Responses to nervous breakdowns in America over a 40-year period. *American Psychologist* 55:740–749.

Tammy. 2000. Personal story of the loss of a multiple. www.angels4ever.com.

Teitelbaum, J. 1996. *From Fatigued to Fantastic*. Garden City Park, New York: Avery.

U.S. Census Bureau. 1998a. *The Official Statistics*, www.census.gov, September 9.

———. 1998b. *Census Bureau Facts for Features*, www.census.gov.

———. 2000. *USA Statistics in Brief—Agriculture, Business, Finance, and Foreign Commerce*, www.census.gov.

U.S. Department of Labor. 1998. *Work and Elder Care: Facts for Caregivers and Their Employers*, www.dol.gov.

U.S. Department of Labor, Bureau of Labor Statistics. 1996. *Consumer Expenditure Survey*, www.dol.gov.

U.S. Department of Labor, Women's Bureau. 1997a. *Black Women in the Labor Force*, www.dol.gov.

———. 1997b. *Women of Hispanic Origin in the Labor Force*, www.dol.gov.

U.S. Department of Transportation. 1999. *Transportation Statistics Annual Report*, www.dot.gov.

Valentine, B. 2000. Personal story of ADHD. www.adhdnews.com.

Weil, A. 1999. Natural help for depression. *Self Healing* September, 1, 6–7.

———. 2000. ADHD: Are we overmedicating children? *Self Healing* August, 8.

Weiss, E. L., J. G. Longhurst, and C. M. Mazure. 1999. Childhood sexual abuse as a risk factor for depression in women: Psychosocial and neurobiological correlates. *Archives of General Psychiatry* 156:816–828.

Weisse, C. S. 1992. Depression and immunocompetence: A review of the literature. *Psychological Bulletin* 111:475–489.

Whelan, K. A. 2000. *Grief Songs: Stories, Letters, and Poems That Chronicle the Recovery and Survival of a Community after the Sudden Death of a Baby*. Boston: Massachusetts Center for Sudden Infant Death Syndrome.

Whiffen, V. E., and I. H. Gotlib. 1989. Infants of postpartum depressed mothers: Temperament and cognitive status. *Journal of Abnormal Psychology* 98:274–279.

Williams, L. M. 1994. Recall of childhood trauma: A prospective study of women's memories of child sexual abuse. *Journal of Consulting & Clinical Psychology* 62:1167–1176.

Wills, J. A. 1937. *The Letters and Speeches of Theodore Roosevelt*. New York: Billington.

Women's Business Network. 2000. Self-employed women. *Working Woman*, November, 4.

Woodbury, R. M. 1925. *Infant Mortality and Its Causes*. Baltimore: Williams and Wilkins.

Working Mother. 2000. Setting up home office. Special Advertising Section. April.

Wright, R. 1997. Go ahead . . . sleep with your children. *APA Monitor,* June, 16–17.

Wurtman, J. J., and S. Suffes. 1997. *The Serotonin Solution to Achieve Permanent Weight Control.* New York: Fawcett Columbine.

Zuravin, S., C. McMillen, D. DePanfilis, and C. Risley-Curtiss. 1996. The intergenerational cycle of child maltreatment: Continuity vs. discontinuity. *Journal of Interpersonal Violence* 11:315–334.

Dr. Kendall-Tackett is a health psycholgist and researcher at the Family Research Lab, University of New Hampshire. She is widely published in the fields of family violence, maternal depression, perinatal health, and disability, and regularly speaks on these topics as well. She works extensively with breastfeeding mothers and is chair of the New Hampshire Breastfeeding Promotion Task Force. She is also a memeber of the Committee on Disability Issues in Psychology, through the American Psychological Association. Her previous book, coauthored with Glenda Kaufman Kantor, is *Postpartum Depression: A Comprehensive Guide for Nurses*, Sage Publications.

Some Other
New Harbinger Titles

Thinking Pregnant, Item TKPG $13.95

Pregnancy Stories, Item PS $14.95

The Co-Parenting Survival Guide, Item CPSG $14.95

Family Guide to Emotional Wellness, Item FGEW $24.95

How to Survive and Thrive in an Empty Nest, Item NEST $13.95

Children of the Self-Absorbed, Item CSAB $14.95

The Adoption Reunion Survival Guide, Item ARSG $13.95

Undefended Love, Item UNLO $13.95

Why Can't I Be the Parent I Want to Be?, Item PRNT $12.95

Kid Cooperation, Item COOP $14.95

Breathing Room: Creating Space to Be a Couple, Item BR $14.95

Why Children Misbehave and What to do About it, Item BEHV $14.95

Couple Skills, Item SKIL $14.95

The Power of Two, Item PWR $15.95

The Queer Parent's Primer, Item QPPM $14.95

Illuminating the Heart, Item LUM $13.95

Dr. Carl Robinson's Basic Baby Care, Item DRR $10.95

The Ten Things Every Parent Needs to Know, Item KNOW $12.95

Healthy Baby, Toxic World, Item BABY $15.95

Becoming a Wise Parent for Your Grown Child, Item WISE $12.95

Stepfamily Realities, Item STEP $16.95

Why are We Still Fighting?, Item FIGH $15.95

Call toll free, **1-800-748-6273,** or log on to our online bookstore **www.newharbinger.com** to order. Have your Visa or Mastercard number ready. Or send a check for the titles you want to New Harbinger Publications, Inc., 5674 Shattuck Ave., Oakland, CA 94609. Include $4.50 for the first book and 75¢ for each additional book, to cover shipping and handling. (California residents please include appropriate sales tax.) Allow two to five weeks for delivery.

Prices subject to change without notice.